You Can
CURE
Yourself

by
Arthur L. Foley II
M.D., Ph.D.

Binford & Mort Publishing

Portland, Oregon 97242

You Can CURE Yourself

Copyright © 1985 by Binford & Mort Publishing

Manufactured in the United States of America.

Library of Congress Catalog Card Number: 85-070166

ISBN: 0-8323-0440-9 (hardcover); 0-8323-0441-7 (softcover)

First Edition 1985

PREFACE

This book is being presented to acquaint the lay public with a viable alternative to the palliative surgical and medical treatment of many of the degenerative diseases. You can *Cure* yourself, if you have the intelligence and the desire.

For the general public, there will be much that is new and perhaps even startling in this work, but there will be nothing that has not been absolutely validated by hard, scientific data. However, some of these data are often overlooked or ignored since they run counter to many of the present and older medical practices and teachings.

It was not until this author suffered a "heart attack" that he became aware of the dramatic relationship between one of these degenerative diseases (coronary heart disease) and the lack of correct nutrition and adequate exercise. This was true despite a medical education and 37 years of medical practice which included a period of time (1963-1978) spent in basic medical research and basic science teaching in two of the country's finest medical schools.

Following the "heart attack", the author began investigating the epidemiology and treatment of coronary heart disease, and thus began a new life-style and a new career in *Nutrition* that finally involved quitting the teaching profession to devote full-time to the study of *Nutrition* and its relationships to disease.

The scientific data supporting these relationships are compelling and the public has but to understand the simple solutions to many of the complex medical problems confronting them today in order to make informed and educated decisions that can be life-saving.

These simple solutions are not easy solutions. They involve a different life-style that changes people's eating habits and their sedentary way of life. However, the patient should always be offered a choice, if one exists, between palliative surgical or medical treatment and the prevention or cure of the disease by correct nutrition.

The diseases and other medical conditions which can be prevented, treated and even cured by correct nutrition and exercise include coronary heart disease, mature-onset diabetes, peptic ulcer and a host of others. We incur these diseases by our carefree eating, drinking and smoking habits and this is often due to a lack of understanding of the damage we are doing to our bodies as a result of years of improper nutrition.

Quite probably every person in the United States is afflicted with one or more of these diseases or medical conditions or has direct knowledge of a family member, relative or friend under treatment. Many people may wish to have a better understanding of one or more of these illnesses, together with some enlightened information regarding prevention, treatment and cure.

This work is designed to explain these diseases in simple language so that all may acquire some basic understanding of each of the illnesses of personal interest and to point out those afflictions which respond to correct nutrition and exercise programs.

May I repeat? Each of us should have a choice, where a choice is feasible, among 3 major treatment modes: palliative surgical treatment such as coronary bypass; palliative medical treatment which often involves hazardous medication; and the preventative, and often curative, treatment with correct nutrition and exercise. The third or curative type of treatment by correct nutrition is seldom offered, it is almost never explained in a simple manner, and it is actually the safest, the most effective and the most economical for the patient.

TABLE OF CONTENTS

LIST OF TABLES

LIST OF ILLUSTRATIONS

INTRODUCTION

Scientists have been studying the epidemiology of disease for centuries and have often noted that the incidence of certain diseases varied with the environment. The causes of many of these illnesses have frequently seemed directly related to diet, and occasionally the lack of a certain vitamin was discovered to explain the malady, or the lack of some mineral was found to play a dominant role in causation. More recently the increased consumption of refined carbohydrates (sugar, white rice and white flour) and the lack of sufficient fiber in the diet have been implicated in the cause, not of just a single disease entity, but of a host of illnesses, many seemingly completely unrelated.

T.L. Cleave and D.P. Burkitt, two brilliant British investigators and scholars, pioneered some work on the relationship of refined carbohydrates and lack of dietary fiber to disease that has made many of us in the medical profession realize that we have seriously neglected the science of *Nutrition*. However, our lack of knowledge in this field is certainly due in part to the fact that the medical profession has never seemed to accept *Nutrition* as a credible discipline and we have been unable to accept or believe what should have been glaringly obvious in our medical practices.

It must be admitted that our medical school training was at fault. *Nutrition* received scant attention and we were taught that medicine and surgery held the ultimate answers to the patients' problems, aided a bit here and there by rather radical and complicated dietary changes, many of which turned out later to be worthless or even harmful.

Many physicians are now acutely aware of the obvious fact that many of the degenerative diseases, and many other maladies as well, are diet and exercise related. These diseases include, among others, the major causes of death from heart disease and many forms of cancer. The scientific evidence is irrefutable. We must educate our patients in *Nutrition*. We should not, as many physicians are accustomed to doing, *assume* that the patients will *not* comply with changes in life-style that involve food, drink and sedentary habits, and so deny them the nutrition education that can be life-saving. Doctors are *not* justified in assuming that no patients have the will-power or moral fiber to save themselves, given the means and the choice.

It is the opinion of this author and many others that physicians must educate the patients in the methods of preventing and curing many of these life-threatening degenerative diseases and many of the less serious ones as well so that each individual can make an educated decision. The patients may either choose to ignore the warnings or they may resolve to avoid the illnesses by changing their life-styles. It is my opinion that all practitioners have the moral responsibility to educate their patients and present them with a choice, if one exists, before taking the easier path of prescribing only palliative medicine or surgery.

Few of us believe that we will die of coronary heart disease or cancer of the bowel, and even fewer realize that proper nutrition and exercise could eliminate the vast majority of these catastrophic illnesses and other diseases as well. If we really care about the future, we can change our life-styles in respect to our eating and exercise habits and look forward to a healthier existence and an extended life-span.

It must be realized however that changing one's life-style is not easy and is not a short-term commitment. Changing one's eating habits to include only those foods that tend to guarantee a healthy future is certainly a difficult task. In many cases it will be comparable to an alcoholic giving up drinking or a drug addict quitting the use of heroin or cocaine. Margaret Mead observed that "one can change religion more easily than food habits."

However, it still amazes some of us that people will submit to open-heart surgery for coronary bypass when correct nutrition and exercise programs can, with more saftey, provide better and longer-lasting benefits. It is also surprising that so many of us endure chronic constipation with the possible grave sequelae of diverticulitis, hemorrhoids and cancer of the colon when correct nutrition could eradicate the problem and prevent the complications. Why do we seem to prefer dangerous medications for high blood pressure when correct nutrition and exercise programs can often prevent or control the hypertension completely? Are these not thought-provoking questions?

Parents are the earliest teachers of nutrition because eating habits and patterns tend to be established early in life. We should therefore begin nutrition education of the parents during pregnancy. It would also seem reasonable to initiate good nutrition practices and education at the preschool, kindergarten and elementary school levels.

Education in nutrition and physical conditioning should be the number one priority of our schools today. Unless our children learn the methods and benefits of correct nutrition and physical conditioning and the damage to health inflicted by poor nutrition, lack of exercise, smoking and drugs, we will continue to be plagued by poor health and the financial burdens incurred by the high costs of medical care for these preventable diseases and practices. Many of the terms used in the following text will be defined as they occur. Some of the more obscure words have been defined or redefined in the glossary.

The author is deeply indebted to the many medical, biological and behavioral scientists who have performed the epidemiological studies, the clinical research, and the basic science research that has made this work possible.

CHAPTER I

Good Nutrition

Human beings are unable to select a nutritionally-sound diet by instinctive reliance on taste and other senses. We require nutrition education and that should begin with a discussion of some of the scientific studies that are bringing to light many environmental factors, especially nutrition and exercise programs, which are exerting major influences in the prevention and curing of certain diseases.

Research has demonstrated unequivocally that there are environmental factors involved in the causation of many forms of cancer and in the production of many degenerative illnesses such as coronary heart disease and cerebrovascular disease. It has been suggested by scientists that perhaps 90% of all cancers may be preventable; and certainly atherosclerosis, the major cause of coronary heart disease and cerebrovascular disease with paralytic stroke, is not only preventable but probably curable, even in some of the later stages.

The dramatic differences in the world-wide distribution of certain diseases has led many people in the research field to investigate the environmental implications of these findings. Breast cancer, for example, has as much lower incidence in Japan than in the United States. However, when the Japanese emigrate to this country, their rate of breast cancer rises. Seventh-Day Adventist vegetarians also have a lower incidence of breast cancer than the rest of the population. The occurrence rate of cancer of the large bowl (colon) has been found to be as much as 10 times higher in some populations, when comparisons are made among peoples of different countries. There are certain

other maladies (peptic ulcer, gall bladder disease, ulcerative colitis and diverticulitis) which are extremely rare or unknown in
the inhabitants of some regions of the world but which are very
common in the industrialized nations.

That certain diseases show such marked differences in prevalence throughout the world, coupled with the evidence that
when people migrate, they and their families become more susceptible, certainly suggests that those illnesses are influenced
by environment and may be preventable.

T.L. Cleave and D.P. Burkitt, brilliant British investigators and
scholars, have made tremendous contributions to the scientific community and to mankind in general by their wide-ranging
epidemiological studies of many diseases, showing the possible relationships of these diseases to environmental factors, especially their associations with dietary differences.

Cleave's observations, investigations and reasoning have led
him to the conclusion that many of the common diseases of
"Western" populations, which are rare in primitive and emerg-
ing cultures, are the result of the increased consumption of
refined food which has, in turn, caused a lack of fiber in the
"Western" diet. This lack of dietary fiber coincides with the
increase in the per capita consumption of refined carbohydrates
(sugar, white rice and white flour). The investigations of Burkitt, and many others in research positions, have tended to con-
firm the validity of many of Cleave's observations and
impressions.

That unrefined carbohydrates with their high fiber content
are important in the prevention and treatment of a host of diseases is now beyond question. Dietary factors are involved in
the production of the three leading causes of death in the United
States today for both men and women. Two-thirds of all deaths
in the Western world populations are due to three illnesses
(coronary heart disease, cancer, and cerebrovascular disease) and
the "Western" diet is a major culprit in the causation of all three.

What is this "Western" diet that we rail against so vehemently,
and that is indicted as the cause of so much of our disease and
suffering? By the "Western" diet, we refer to the prevailing diet
consumed in the developed countries of the "Western" world,
such as the United States and Europe. This diet is high in refined
carbohydrates and fats and therefore tends to be low in fiber.

When one considers that fiber is the undigestible portion of the cell walls of fruits, vegetables, legumes and whole grains, and that refined sugar, meat, fats, oils and dairy products contain no fiber at all, it becomes abundantly clear that many of us are choosing most of our food from the fiber-free groups. Fiber must be obtained by eating fruits, vegetables, legumes, whole grain cereals, and whole grain breads.

Fiber, in order to perform its necessary functions well, apparently must be taken in a natural state, not as an additive sprinkled on food. When there is sufficient fiber in one's diet, the weight and bulk of the bowel movement in increased, the consistency of the stool becomes softer and more normal, intraluminal pressure against the bowel wall in decreased causing less damage to the lining, and the transit time through the colon is decreased, providing less contact time for noxious substances as they progress through the gut tract.

Lack of fiber in the diet tends to result in long intestinal transit time, increase in the intraluminal pressures, and small hard stools that are often difficult to pass.

400 years before Christ, Hippocrates, the Father of Medicine, observed the value of a high fiber diet as a laxative and dietary promoter of health. He did not know what fiber was, but his keen observations and deductive reasoning convinced him that diet and health were inextricably bound. He urged the citizens of Athens to "eat whole-meal bread, fruits and vegetables to ensure large, bulky bowel movements of easy passage" as an important step in preventative medicine.

Why don't the modern doctors teach their patients the importance of good nutrition? Why does today's physician stress drugs or surgery as the answer to the many medical problems which can be much better and more safely treated by a correct nutritional program? Four answers to these questions come to mind immediately. First, the doctor's training was at fault. Until very recently, little or no nutrition was included in the medical curriculum; and even now, some medical schools teach no formal courses in this most important discipline. Second, it is much easier and quicker to prescribe a drug or surgery than to teach the patients how to change their life-styles as regards their eating habits. Third, the physicians will probably claim that it is impossible to get their patients to comply with dietary advice so, rather than waste valuable time and effort, they feel obligated to recommend palliative treatment in the form of drugs and surgery, rather than the curative measures. Fourth, the patients often will not believe that a change in their eating, drinking and smoking habits can possibly be as effective as the new miracle drugs or exotic surgery. They would rather seek out a doctor who will allow them some of their "pet" addictions such as alcohol, cigarettes, caffeine, simple sugars, fat and greasy fried foods. They may insist on a physician who will substitute palliative drugs and surgery for some temporary relief, rather than one who will demand that they learn something about nutrition and make some of the difficult changes in life-style that can bring about a cure.

Let us take, for example, patients who have had palliative surgery, such as coronary bypass. Do you think that coronary bypass cures anyone? Of course it doesn't. They may feel more comfortable, secure and confident, but diseased arteries are still there with the most narrowed portions bypassed. The patients' arteries will continue to narrow and clog, and the bypass vessels as well, if they don't change their life-styles and get on a correct nutrition regimen and a carefully-monitored exercise program, specifically tailored to their unique situations. These are the curative presciptions that involve drastic changes in life-style, but which would have made the palliative bypass surgery unnecessary.

Education of the patient in preventative medicine is probably the most important responsibility of the physician, but this has not always been appreciated by many of us. Some of the benefits of good nutrition on many aspects of health have been understood for centuries, but only relatively recently has it become so apparent that so many of the most seriously disabling medical problems, including the major diseases involved in the three leading causes of death in the United States today, can be prevented by correct nutrition.

All of us, especially our little children, should learn the nutrition fundamentals of preventative medicine. Our concerns should not be calories or supplemental vitamins and minerals, but which foods and which methods of preparation can, in the majority of cases, practically guarantee improved health and increased life-expectancy.

We have gathered together a group of diseases, many seemingly completely unrelated, which respond phenomenally well to treatment with the combination of correct nutrition and regular, judicious physical exercise. Many are completely preventable, many are curable, and all are immeasurably benefitted by these programs.

CHAPTER II

Correct Nutrition

"Correct nutrition" is always good nutrition, but good nutrition is not necessarily synonymous with correct nutrition. "Correct nutrition" is a type of nutrition regimen which is specially designed to protect your health. It combines both preventative and curative features. If you follow the simple rules listed below, you will certainly improve your health, the quality of your life, and your life-expectancy.

1. Eat as much cereal as you wish, but choose only those cereals listed. Use nothing on the cereal except skim milk and raisins or some other fruit.

2. Eat as much fresh, raw, natural fruit as you like. You may also eat dried fruit, but eat only those listed. Eat no canned fruits which contain chemical additives or preservatives even though most of these additives and preservatives are probably perfectly safe.

3. Eat all the fresh, natural vegetables and legumes that you wish. Most of the vegetables should preferably be eaten raw or steamed, but they may be boiled. Eat no processed, packaged or canned vegetables with chemical additives or preservatives even though these additives and preservatives may consist only of sugars and salt.

4. Eat as much soup as you may desire but only the home-made variety consisting of peas, beans, barley and fresh vegetables chosen from the lists.

5. Eat broiled or baked meat or fish no more than four times each week and no more than four ounces at one meal. Choose only meats listed.

6. Eat as much boiled brown rice as you wish, but add nothing but salsa, meats from the list, or fresh natural vegetables.

7. Eat all the bread desired if it is whole-wheat bread or whole-wheat pocket-bread with no chemical additives or preservatives such as added sugars, honey or fats.

8. Eat as much fresh fruit and fresh vegetable salad as you wish. No salad dressings are allowed, especially fats and oils.

9. Sandwiches—Tuna, chicken or turkey with lettuce, celery, and other fresh vegetables make wonderful sandwich fillers. Slices of banana in toasted pocket-bread is a favorite of many.

10. Postum is a marvelous substitute for coffee or tea after one gets used to it, and it is caffeine free. Skim milk is another good nutritious drink. It is high in protein and calcium content and is especially good for pregnant women. It is also especially good for menopausal women, postmenopausal women and all elderly persons to prevent the bone-thinning and weakening of osteoporosis.

11. One further and most important announcement—you must get your fiber from natural fruits, vegetables, legumes and whole-grain cereals and breads.

There are a few dietary restrictions which bear constant emphasis, repetition and strictly-defined descriptions:

1. No refined carbohydrates (sugar, white rice, white flour) or products made with refined sugars and flour such as cookies, cakes, etc.

2. No poultry skin.

3. No cooking oil or salad dressing oil.

4. No excess fat (fat should be trimmed from beef or broiled away from hamburger).

5. No honey, molasses, syrups, jams, jellies, etc. Use only fruits for sweeteners.

6. No butter, margarine, oils, sauces, dressings or gravies.

7. No fried foods and no cooking oil.

8. No processed or packaged foods if feasible, especially if they contain chemical additives or preservatives even though these additives and preservatives may be perfectly safe such as sugar and salt.

9. No cigarette smoking.

10. No alcohol if your nutrition regimen is to be absolutely correct.

11. No caffeine such as coffee, tea, cocoa, chocolate, or caffeine-containing soft drinks.

The above rules define a good and a correct nutrition regimen. Unlimited food and calories can be chosen from the following food lists except for the few restrictions mentioned above such as four ounces of meat only four meals per week and nothing from the "Foods to Avoid" list which is included only to point out what damage you can inflict on yourself with some of the more common aberrations from good nutrition practices. These include the use of oils in cooking, salad dressings and the consumption of ice cream. Remember what Margaret Mead observed, "it is easier to change religion than one's eating habits." This nutrition regimen will not be easy for the first few weeks, but after that you will come to accept it and actually may come to like it.

If we follow this nutrition regimen, we will not need to worry about vitamin or mineral supplements. All will be provided. Calories will be no problem either. Your weight will be maintained at a normal level or begin to slowly fall toward that level. Of course, excessive fat will disappear more rapidly if you choose the lower-calorie foods, but a correct nutrition regimen is designed mainly as a change in life-style and a method of maintaining or regaining health. Rapid weight loss can be accomplished on this regimen (see Chapter IV on Obesity), but that is an entirely different story.

The Food Lists

The following food lists include the acceptable fruits and berries, the vegetables, legumes and seeds, the meats and skim milk, the fish, the breads and cereals. One should choose food only from these lists and should try to follow the simple rules enumerated at the beginning of this chapter. There should be no restriction on either the quantity or variety of foods consumed from these lists except for the meats and fish. Fruits, berries and vegetables should be chosen from the fresh produce counters if possible. Many of the vegetables would be better eaten raw and these include broccoli, cabbage, carrots, cauliflower, celery, cucumbers, lettuce, onions, parsnips, sweet green peppers, radishes, rutabaga, summer squash, tomatoes and turnips. If cooking is desired, the best method would be steaming which preserves vitamins and minerals. The only other acceptable methods of food preparation should be boiling, broiling or baking. Nothing should be fried or cooked in oil or grease.

Foods are composed of *Protein, Fat, Carbohydrates* (sugars and starches), *fiber, minerals, vitamins* and *water.* Each food is listed in Column 1 of Table II-1, and each is then described in Columns 2 through 8 to provide the reader with some rather detailed information. For example, if one wishes to know the caloric value of a food, consult Column 2 which lists the number of calories in 100 grams or 3-1/2 ounces of the edible portion of that food. Column 3 lists the caloric value of the protein content of 100 grams or 3-1/2 ounces of that food so that we may easily pick out foods with high or low protein content. Columns 4 through 8 similarly list the values or amounts of some of the more important constituents of each food so that we may easily and quickly locate foods with high calcium content, high iron content, high fiber content, etc.

The proteins and carbohydrates in foods yield approximately 4 calories from each gram. Therefore, if 100 grams (3-1/2 ounces) of cabbage yield 4 calories from its protein content, there must be about 1 gram of protein in 100 grams of cabbage. If 100 grams of cabbage yield 36 calories from its carbohydrate constituents, it must contain about 9 grams of carbohydrate. Fat however yields approximately 9 calories from each gram, so 100 grams of cabbage must contain very little fat, only 2/9 of a gram.

To explain Table II-1 once more, let us go down Column 1 and pick, for example, blackberries. Column 2 tells us that there are 52 calories in 100 grams (3-1/2 ounces) of raw blackberries. Column 3 shows us that 3 of those calories come from protein. Column 4 indicates that 3 of the calories come from fat, and Column 5 that the remaining 46 calories derive from carbohydrate (complex sugars and starches). Column 6 indicates that blackberries are high in fiber content, and Column 7 and 8 give us the milligrams of calcium and iron, respectively, in 100 grams or 3-1/2 ounces.

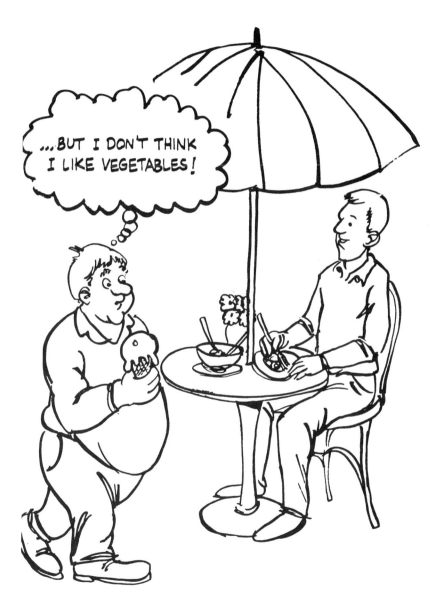

ILLUSTRATION II-I

TABLE II-1

Column 1	Column 2	Column 3	Column 4	Column 5	Column 6	Column 7	Column 8
Food	Calories/100gm Edible Portion	Calories from Protein	Calories from Fat	Calorie from CHO	Grams of Fiber	Milligrams of Calcium	Milligrams of Iron
FRUITS AND BERRIES							
Apples (raw)	58	1	5	52	0.77	7.	0.18
One apple (3/lb or 150 grams)	80	1	7	72	—	—	—
One apple (4/lb or 115 grams)	61	1	5	55	—	—	—
Applesauce (canned unsweetened)	43	0	0	43	0.53	3.	0.1
Apricots (raw)	48	5	3	40	0.6	14.	0.54
Apricots (dehydrated)	320	17	5	298	2.95	61.	6.31
Avocado (raw)	161	7	128	26	2.11	11.	1.02
Banana (raw)	92	4	4	84	0.5	6.	0.31
Blackberries (raw)	52	3	3	46	4.1	32.	0.57
Blueberries (raw)	56	2	3	51	1.3	6.	0.17

Cherries (sour, red, raw)	50	3	3	44	0.2	16.	0.32
Cherries (sweet, raw)	72	4	8	59	0.4	15.	0.39
Dates (domestic natural, dry)	275	7	4	264	2.2	32.	1.15
Figs (dried and uncooked)	255	10	10	235	4.8	144.	2.23
Grapefruit (raw)	32	2	1	29	0.2	12.	0.06
Grapefruit juice (unsweetened, canned, raw)	36	2	1	33	0.0	9.	0.2
Grapes (slip-skin, raw)	65	2	3	60	0.76	14.	0.29
Grapes (adherent skin, raw)	71	2	5	64	0.45	11.	0.26
Melons, cantaloupe (raw)	35	3	2	30	0.36	11.	0.21
Melons, casaba (raw)	26	3	1	22	0.5	5.	0.4
Melons, honeydew (raw)	35	1	1	33	0.6	6.	0.07
Oranges (raw)	47	3	1	43	0.43	40.	0.1

TABLE II-1—Continued

Column 1 Food	Column 2 Calories/100gm Edible Portion	Column 3 Calories from Protein	Column 4 Calories from Fat	Column 5 Calorie from CHO	Column 6 Grams of Fiber	Column 7 Milligrams of Calcium	Column 8 Milligrams of Iron
FRUITS AND BERRIES—continued							
Orange juice (squeezed)	45	2	2	41	0.1	11.	0.2
Peaches (raw)	43	2	1	40	0.64	5.	0.11
Peaches (dehydrated)	325	16	7	302	3.97	38.0	5.51
Peaches (dried)	239	2	6	231	2.93	28.0	4.06
Pears (raw)	59	1	3	55	1.4	11.0	0.25
Pineapple (raw)	49	1	4	44	0.54	7.	0.37
Pineapple juice (canned)	56	1	1	54	0.1	17.	0.26
Plums (raw)	55	3	5	47	0.6	4.	0.1
Prunes (dried, uncooked)	239	9	4	226	2.04	51.	2.48
Raisins (seeded)	296	8	5	283	1.28	28.	2.59

Raspberries (raw)	49	3	4	42	3.0	22.	0.57
Strawberries (raw)	30	2	3	25	0.53	14.	0.38
Tangerines	44	2	2	40	0.33	14.	0.1
Watermelon	32	2	4	26	0.3	8.	0.17

VEGETABLES, LEGUMES AND SEEDS

Asparagus	26	8	2	16	0.7	22.	1.0
Barley	350	28	1	321	0.5	16.	2.0
Beans (Great Northern) (dry)	340	76	14	260	1.5	144.	8.0
Beans (Green Snap) (raw)	32	6	2	24	1.0	56.	0.8
Beans (Lima) (dry)	123	29	4	90	1.8	72.	7.8
Beans (Pea, Navy,) (dry)	340	74	14	252	1.5	144.	8.0
Beans (Yellow, Wax) (raw)	27	6	2	19	1.0	56.	0.8
Beets (peeled, raw)	43	5	1	37	0.8	16.	0.7
Beet Greens (raw)	18	6	2	10	1.1	118.	3.3
Broccoli	32	12	2	18	1.5	103.	1.1
Brussel Sprouts	45	16	2	27	1.6	36.	1.5

TABLE II-1—Continued

Column 1 Food	Column 2 Calories/100gm Edible Portion	Column 3 Calories from Protein	Column 4 Calories from Fat	Column 5 Calorie from CHO	Column 6 Grams of Fiber	Column 7 Milligrams of Calcium	Column 8 Milligrams of Iron
VEGETABLES, LEGUMES AND SEEDS—continued							
Buckwheat Flour (whole-grain)	335	47	2	286	9.9	32.	2.7
Cabbage	24	4	2	18	0.8	50.	0.4
Carrots	42	4	2	36	1.0	37.	0.7
Cauliflower	27	9	2	16	1.0	25.	1.1
Celery	17	3	1	13	0.6	40.	0.3
Chard, Swiss	18	6	1	11	0.8	90.	3.2
Chick Peas or Garbanzos	360	70	45	245	5.0	150.	6.9
Collard (leaves and no stems)	45	16	7	22	1.2	203.	1.0
Corn, Sweet (on cob)	53	7	4	42	0.7	1.5	0.3
Cowpeas or Blackeye (dry, immature)	127	31	2	89	1.8	27.	2.3

Food							
Cowpeas or Blackeye (dry, mature)	343	48	11	285	4.4	74.	6.0
Cucumbers	15	3	1	11	0.6	25.	1.1
Eggplant, cooked	19	3	2	14	0.9	11.	0.6
Endive	20	6	1	13	0.9	80.	1.7
Kale	53	20	7	26	1.3	—	—
Lentils (dry mature seeds)	340	84	10	246	3.9	80.	6.8
Lettuce	13	3	1	9	0.5	35.	2.0
Mushrooms	28	11	2	15	0.8	6.	0.8
Okra	36	8	2	26	1.0	92.	0.6
Onions	38	5	1	32	0.6	27.	0.5
Parsnips	76	5	4	67	2.0	42.5	0.6
Peas (dry, mature, split) (no seed coat)	348	83	9	257	1.2	33.	5.1
Peppers (raw, sweet)	22	4	2	16	1.4	9.0	0.7
Potatoes (pared before cooking and boiled)	65	6	1	58	0.5	6.0	0.5

TABLE II-1—Continued

Column 1	Column 2	Column 3	Column 4	Column 5	Column 6	Column 7	Column 8
Food	Calories/100gm Edible Portion	Calories from Protein	Calories from Fat	Calorie from CHO	Grams of Fiber	Milligrams of Calcium	Milligrams of Iron
VEGETABLES, LEGUMES AND SEEDS—continued							
Potatoes (pared, raw)	76	7	1	68	0.5	7.0	0.6
Pumpkin (canned)	33	3	3	27	1.1	25.	0.4
Radishes	17	3	1	13	0.7	30.	1.0
Rhubarb (raw)	13	3	1	9	0.7	96.	0.82
Rice, brown	360	26	17	317	0.9	32.	1.6
Rutabaga	35	3	1	31	1.1	59.	0.3
Sesame Seeds	563	67	411	85	6.3	110.	2.4
Soybeans (dry, mature)	403	116	158	129	4.9	226.	8.4
Spaghetti (dry, unenriched)	369	43	11	315	0.3	27.	1.3
Spinach	26	11	3	12	0.6	93.	3.1

Squash (raw, summer)	19	4	1	14	0.6	28.	0.4
Squash (raw, winter) acorn, butternut, hubbard)	40	4	1	35	1.4	28.	0.8
Sunflower Seeds (dry, hulled)	560	82	420	58	3.8	120.	7.0
Sweet Potatoes (boiled in skin, no skin)	114	6	4	104	0.7	32.	0.7
Tomatoes (raw)	20	3	2	15	0.5	12.	0.5
Turnips (raw)	23	3	2	18	0.9	40.	0.5
Yams (raw)	87	6	2	79	0.9	17.	0.5
MEATS AND MILK							
Beef (ground, 10% fat)	173	83	90	0	0.0	12.	3.1
Beef (dried, chipped)	194	137	57	0	0.0	20.	5.1
Chicken (roasted, meat only)	190	123	67	0	0.0	24.	1.39
Chicken (stewed)	177	117	60	0	0.0	14.	1.17

TABLE II-1—Continued

Column 1	Column 2	Column 3	Column 4	Column 5	Column 6	Column 7	Column 8
Food	Calories/100gm Edible Portion	Calories from Protein	Calories from Fat	Calorie from CHO	Grams of Fiber	Milligrams of Calcium	Milligrams of Iron
MEATS AND MILK—continued							
Chicken (raw, light meat with no skin)	114	99	15	0	0.0	12.	0.73
Chicken (roasted, light meat with no skin)	173	132	41	0	0.0	15.	1.06
Chicken (raw, dark meat with no skin)	125	86	39	0	0.0	12.	1.03
Chicken (roasted, dark meat with no skin)	205	117	88	0	0.0	15.0	1.33
Egg White	49	44	0	5	0.0	9.	0.11
Milk, Skim	35	13	2	20	0.0	121.	0.04
Turkey (raw, flesh only, no skin)	119	93	26	0	0.0	12.	1.44

Turkey (roasted, flesh only, no skin)	170	125	45	0	0.0	20.	1.96
Turkey (raw, light meat, no skin)	115	86	39	0	0.0	10.	1.22
Turkey (roasted, light meat, no skin)	157	128	29	0	0.0	15.	1.57
Turkey (raw, dark meat, no skin)	125	85	40	0	0.0	13.	1.66
Turkey roasted, dark meat, no skin)	187	122	65	0	0.0	26.	2.41
Venison (raw and lean)	124	88	36	0	0.0	10.6	—
FISH							
Cod	162	114	48	0	0.0	31.	1.0
Salmon (Atlantic)	203	93	110	0	0.0	—	—
Salmon (Chinook, King)	211	85	126	0	0.0	154.	0.9
Salmon (Coho, Silver)	153	89	64	0	0.0	244.	0.9
Scallops (steamed)	112	99	13	0	0.0	115.	3.0

TABLE II-1—Continued

Column 1	Column 2	Column 3	Column 4	Column 5	Column 6	Column 7	Column 8
Food	Calories/100gm Edible Portion	Calories from Protein	Calories from Fat	Calorie from CHO	Grams of Fiber	Milligrams of Calcium	Milligrams of Iron
FISH—continued							
Tuna (packed in water)	127	120	7	0	0.0	16.	1.6
BREADS, MACARONI AND SPAGHETTI							
Bread (wholewheat) 1 Slice (whole-wheat)	243	42	27	174	1.6-2.1	99.	3.0
Crackers (saltines)	81	14	9	58	.05-.07	33.	1.0
Cracker (one saltine)	432	31	107	294	0.4	20.8	1.2
Macaroni (dry, unenriched)	12	1	3	8	—	—	—
Spaghetti (dry, unenriched)	370	50	11	309	0.3	27.	1.3
	369	43	11	315	0.3	27.	1.3

CEREALS

All Bran	249	26	15	208	36.9	81.	15.9
40% Bran Flakes	326	36	16	274	17.6	49.	28.6
Corn Grits (dry)	371	30	10	331	2.1	2.	3.91
Cream of Wheat	370	42	13	315	2.2	141.	28.6
Grapenuts	357	43	0	314	4.8	38.	4.34
Oatmeal (Quaker and Fortified)	369	54	51	254	1.1	576.	22.28

FOODS TO BE AVOIDED

Butter	716	2	712	2	0.0	20.	0.0
Egg	158	52	101	5	0.0	54.	2.3
Fats, cooking (vegetable fat and mixed fat shortening)	900	0	900	0	0.0	0.0	0.0
Honey	304	1	0	303	—	5.	0.5
Ice Cream (vanilla; rich hardened)	236	10	144	82	0.0	146.	0.06

TABLE II-1—Continued

Column 1	Column 2	Column 3	Column 4	Column 5	Column 6	Column 7	Column 8
Food	Calories/100gm Edible Portion	Calories from Protein	Calories from Fat	Calorie from CHO	Grams of Fiber	Milligrams of Calcium	Milligrams of Iron
FOODS TO BE AVOIDED—continued							
Ice Cream (soft serve)	218	16	117	85	0.0	146.	0.06
Margarine	720	2	716	2	0.0	20.	0.0
Mayonnaise (salad dressing)	390	4	295	91	0.0	18.	0.5
Molasses (medium)	232	—	—	232	—	290.	6.0
Peanut Butter	590	100	454	36	1.8	59.	1.9
Sherbet	140	4	16	120	0.0	16.	trace
Sugar, white (granulated)	385	0	0	385	0.0	0.0	0.1
Sugar, brown	373	0	0	373	0.0	85.	3.4
Syrup, Cane	263	0	0	263	0.0	60.	3.6
Syrup, Maple	252	—	—	252	—	104.	1.2

Syrup (table blends)	290	0	0	290	0.0	46.	4.1
Sorghum	257	—	—	257	—	172.	12.5
Yogurt, plain (whole milk)	61	14	28	19	0.0	111.	0.4

Alcoholic Drinks	Approximate Calories
Ale (8 oz.)	98
Beer (12 oz.)	150
Wine (4 oz.)	100
Gin (1½ oz.)	104-133
Scotch (1½ oz.)	104-133
Vodka (1½ oz.)	104-133
Whiskey (1½ oz.)	104-133

CHAPTER III

Exercise Program

Regular, relatively strenuous physical exercise and good nutrition are the two major prerequisites for the full enjoyment of the "good life". An exercise program that is tailored to the unique needs of the individual will improve the health, the quality and the length of life.

If we ignore that aphorism, it is only a matter of time until the degenerative diseases begin to take their toll. Genetic and environmental differences will cause some to develop these diseases early in life, while others seem to remain relatively immune for years, but all are debauched before their time if they disregard those basic tenets.

Do you believe that exercise is only for the foolish and other assorted "exhibitionists" and "nuts"? If this is your attitude, this section is "must" reading. Most people are not aware that constant changes are going on in their bodies at all times. They don't realize that dynamic growth, absorption and realignment of cells is occurring unremittingly in all tissues and organs at all ages. Body cells are dying constantly and replacement processes are at work and, if we don't create a need for muscle and bone strength, etc., the structures undergoing disuse will deteriorate. "If you don't use it, you lose it."

What are the vascular consequences when we neglect daily, reasonably strenuous physical exercise and ingest a gourmet diet? The answer is simple. We begin to clog our arteries with a slow but inexorable build-up of atheromatous plaque. This then may bring on every degenerative disease discussed in this book and many are life-threatening or even absolutely deadly.

As the coronary arteries nourishing the heart become narrow and clogged, we become candidates for angina pectoris (exertional chest pain), myocardial infarction and "sudden death". As the arteries supplying the brain become narrowed by the atherosclerotic plaque, we become subject to cerebral thrombosis, "stroke" and senility. Blockage of arteries to the kidneys can produce high blood pressure and kidney failure. Atheromatous plaque, impeding the blood supply to the legs and feet, brings on intermittent claudication (severe leg pains on walking) progressing to cold, pulseless feet. Further deterioration of the blood supply may then cause necrotic leg and foot ulcers and even gangrene requiring amputation. And that, unfortunately, isn't even all of the atherosclerosis "horror" story.

This is what happens to your body when you neglect regular, reasonably strenuous physical exercise, and lapse into a sedentary life-style. All atherosclerotic arterial disease begins to progress more rapidly, and you become at risk of coronary heart disease, "stroke", etc. Your muscle mass and strength deteriorate and your bones undergo osteoporosis, making them more susceptible to fracture. Did you know, if your leg were to be immobilized in a plaster cast for two months, that the bones of your leg would undergo osteoporotic changes with thinning and weakening of the bone structure? Do you realize that those unused leg muscles would be weakened and deteriorated to the point where you could actually see the reduced circumference of the leg that had been immobilized when compared to the normal one? What if you then tried to walk? You would find that the joints had become stiff, there would be marked limitation of joint movement, and aching and pain would be present along with the muscle weakness. Anyone who has suffered a broken leg can testify to this. These same phenomena occur with the sedentary life-style, but they often come on so gradually that we don't realize they are happening until we try to throw a ball or get ready for a ski trip. We decide that "age" must be creeping up on us. It isn't "age" so much as lack of regular, reasonably strenuous physical activity.

Many people are content to "stiffen up", to be unable to make a fist because their fingers won't bend far enough, and to "shuffle about" because it is too painful to stride along in an upright position. As they move less and less, they tend to become more and more stiff, and severe limitation of motion may finally make them almost complete invalids. Do you think that a few rounds of golf each week or a tennis game every Saturday morning can substitute for regular, reasonably strenuous physical activity? If you do, you are only deluding yourself and ensuring that the degenerative diseases will inexorably do you in. You must decide whether or not you want the degenerative diseases with their miserable often life-threatening consequences to complicate and inevitably shorten your life. You can escape many of the "horrors", if you can learn to get by without cigarettes, eat the nutritionally-sound diet, and exercise relatively strenuously and *daily*, "come hell or high water". You owe it to yourself and perhaps to those who love you.

You should walk two miles in 30 minutes or less, seven days a week.

Exercise Program
(50 years of age or older)

Regular, reasonably strenuous physical activity is a "must" if you intend to maintain a healthy body and mind and avoid the degenerative diseases and senility. Remember that *regular* means *daily*.

Walking is the best physical activity, but if for some reason you are unable to walk, you are probably going to need professional advice in order to ensure that you bring specific muscles into play. Be certain that weight-bearing occurs to prevent osteoporosis, that arms and legs are both involved in the activity to prevent "disuse atrophy" of muscles and be sure that the exercise stresses your cardiovascular system (heart and blood vessels) to keep it healthy.

Weight-bearing is necessary to prevent osteoporosis (bone thinning and weakening) which is responsible for so many fractures, especially in postmenopausal women. Osteoporosis is extremely common in both sexes after age 50 and is the rule after age 70. It is aggravated by hormone deficiency in women, but its main causes are lack of regular, relatively strenuous physical activity and too little emphasis on including high calcium foods in the diet. The arms and legs must be forcefully activated daily to prevent "joint stiffness", limitation of motion and dis-use atrophy of muscles and to foster good circulation of blood through the arteries supplying the arms and legs. The cardiovas-cular system (heart and blood vessels) must be stressed to pre-vent atherosclerosis, especially the atherosclerotic narrowing and clogging of the arteries nourishing the heart and brain.

How far and how fast you should walk each day depends on a great many factors. Should a medical person design your pro-gram, or does your physician think that your health is good enough that you can design your own, given the following guidelines?

1. Walk once a day for the specific purpose of preventing atherosclerosis and fulfilling the requirements of your exercise program. *You must walk twice each day* if you are being *treated* for atherosclerotic *heart disease, adult-onset diabetes* or *atherosclerotic senile changes.*

2. Carry a walking stick, riding crop or an umbrella to ward off obstreperous dogs and to exercise your fingers, hands and forearms.

3. Start your walking program by walking quite leisurely until you can walk 2 miles easily. Then, begin timing yourself and gradually increase the speed until you can walk 2 miles in 30 minutes.

4. Wear comfortable, good quality jogging or running shoes and rather heavy tube socks.

5. Walk inside in inclement weather. A shopping mall or gym will often serve nicely.

6. Practice carrying your weight a bit forward so that you do not come down hard on your heels with each step. Hitting hard on your heels jars and pounds your joints and can lead to problems in your back, hips and knees. Try to learn to pull your-self forward a bit with your toes thus strengthening the foot, leg and thigh muscles and avoiding the shock to joints.

7. If you are able to jog, you may need only 20 minutes or less for your 2-mile daily work-out.

    (a.) *Don't jog* if you are excessively fat or obese. Wait until you attain a normal weight, because you may damage your joints by jogging, and walking is just as good for you.

    (b.) *Don't jog* until your foot muscles and calf muscles are

strong enough to allow you to run comfortably on
your toes for at least 200 meters because, if your muscles tire too soon, jogging can shock your joints
excessively.

(c.) It is hazardous to run or jog without allowing the heels
to touch the ground unless you are in excellent condition; because tendonitis, inflammation of the
Achilles tendon, may occur and disable you for weeks.

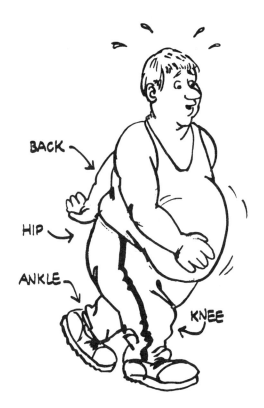

DON'T JOG IF YOU ARE OVERWEIGHT!
YOU'LL RUIN YOUR JOINTS.

ILLUSTRATION III-1

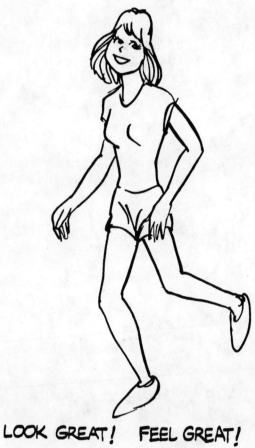

LOOK GREAT!   FEEL GREAT!

ILLUSTRATION III-2

CHAPTER IV

Obesity

Obesity means excessively fat; and this condition is so prevalent and constitutes such a tremendous health hazard that it has become one of the most critical problems facing the medical profession today. In any culture where refined carbohydrates (sugar, white rice and white flour) are abundant and easily obtainable, and where a sedentary life-style is the rule, many individuals will be overweight and many will be obese. Excessive accumulation of fat will inevitably occur in any healthy individual whenever the caloric intake exceeds the requirements for maintenance of body functions and physcial activity.

Eating habits are generally fixed at an early age, and where family and cultural influences place great emphasis on food there is a marked tendency to establish a pattern of overeating early in life.

In a few obese patients, a glandular disorder such as hypothyroidism or hypopituitarism may be a significant factor in causing excessive weight gain. In other overweight individuals, a derangement of the "appetite control centers" in the hypothalamic portion of the brain may be at fault. If one's hypothalamic set-point for appetite control is too high or abnormally low, the desire for more or less food than needed may become a major determinant of the state of obesity or thinness. There are also overweight persons with psychological problems, and these individuals may substitute food for the satisfaction they should be receiving from other emotional sources such as family, friends, business and hobbies.

However, the vast majority of us, who now have or in the past have had the problem of obesity, are probably addicted to certain kinds of foods. Our cravings for these foods resemble the dependencies of the cigarette fiends, the alcoholics and the drug addicts. The obese individuals may need their "fix" in the form of sugar-rich food or fat, almost as desperately as the cigarette fiends require their cigarettes, the alcoholics their beer, wine or whiskey, and the drug addicts their heroin or cocaine. Many of us are undoubtedly "food-aholics", and if we cannot at least admit this to ourselves, our situations are possibly hopeless.

Some of the dangers of obesity are dramatically illustrated in the morbidity and mortality statistics from many of the medical disciplines. It is dangerous to give general anesthetics to markedly overweight people, and surgical mortality studies demonstrate the increased risks involved in operative procedures performed on the obese, and we could go on and on.

As one might reasonably expect, because the type of diet is often the major factor in causation, obesity is closely associated with many of the degenerative diseases, especially atherosclerotic coronary heart disease, arthritis and diabetes; and the treatment of these maladies includes the same nutrition program as that used to remedy the excessive accumulation of fat. It is also true that obesity is a major contributing factor in all of the common causes of death.

When the obese or overweight individuals finally make their decision to lose their unwanted fat and then remain at a desired or pleasing weight, they should be aware that a change in life-style will be necessary for success and that a long-term commitment must be made and honored. Many of us lack the willpower to do more than lose a few pounds and then revert to our old eating habits that got us into trouble in the first place. But for those of us with the will power to persist to success like the reformed cigarette smokers, alcoholics and drug addicts who recognize their dependencies, there is but one option. We must make a long-term commitment to a change in life-style and then go about the business of losing weight in a slow, safe, sensible and healthful manner. One should first set a specified goal that is realistic, and then should calculate how many months or years might be reasonably needed to attain the goal. If one is 50 pounds overweight, it would be realistic to plan on losing one pound per week for one year. If individuals are 100 pounds overweight and decide to lose the 100 pounds in one year, they may expect problems, because averaging a two-pound weight loss for 50 consecutive weeks can be extremely difficult and very hard on a good disposition.

Persons intending to lose weight must realize that while they may not have to limit the quantity of food eaten, they will need to choose their foods from the prescribed lists and keep their caloric intake 3500 calories per week below their *Maintenance Level* in order to lose one pound of body fat per week, and 7000 calories below in order to lose two pounds of body fat. At this point, it might be well to admonish you that "if food tastes very, very good, it is very, very likely to be bad for you". That is of course not entirely true, but it will seem distressingly so when one begins thinking of candy, sugar, honey, cookies, cakes, deep-fried foods and marbled steaks. When you study the food lists, you may think that this is no diet at all, and actually it is not a diet in the sense that diets are usually very restrictive of both variety and quantity. On this weight-loss program, you will get all of the protein, fats, carbohydrates and fiber that you need and more. You will also receive plenty of vitamins and minerals; and if you wish to lose excess weight more rapidly at any time, just decrease the amounts of the higher-calorie foods in favor of some of the lower-calorie items.

The first and most important fact to be considered in any weight reduction program is the cause of obesity. Why are we excessively fat? If we don't have a clear and complete understanding of the reason, how can we hope to solve the problem?

Let's face it. We are fat, not because of the quantity we consume but because we eat too much sugar and fat. We overeat because we may ingest a thousand calories or more of sugar and fat without feeling "full" or satisfied. The calories in our fried and sugary foods are too concentrated and lack the bulk or fiber which can tell us when we should stop eating, that we have ingested an adequate amount of food. If we ate only fresh vegetables and fruits, legumes, sugar-free cereals and whole-grain breads and skim milk, we would feel "full" or satiated long before we had consumed any great excess of calories. Sugar, honey, candy, syrups, jam, jelly, butter, peanut butter, cake, cookies, sweet rolls, fried and greasy foods, deep-fried foods, ice cream, whole milk, marbled steaks, etc., give us packed calories but insufficient bulk to properly satisfy our appetites, so we tend to continue ingesting more and more calories in excess of our body requirements. Our body tends to react correctly to bulky, fiber-rich foods and tells us when we are satiated or "full". So, why are we fat? Simply because we eat too much sugar and fat instead of the bulky, fiber-rich fresh fruits and vegetables, legumes and sugar-free cereals and whole-grain breads. It is as simple as that.

The second lesson in a weight reduction course should involve simple arithmetic. We must understand that food contains calories, and that 3500 excess calories, above those needed to maintain body function and normal daily activity, will add one pound of fat to our body and 7000 calories, two pounds. To lose two pounds of body fat, we must take in 7000 calories less than is needed for body maintenance. The calorie maintenance requirements for body weight and functions vary with the size of the individual, the amount of work performed or energy expended, the environmental conditions, etc. The 130 pound persons who lead sedentary existences in warm surroundings may need only 1500 calories per day to maintain their weight, but if they were forced to perform hard, manual labor in sub-freezing weather, they might require 6000 calories or more per day to prevent weight loss. Your *"Maintenance Level"* can be defined as the caloric intake that maintains your weight without significant gain or loss as you carry out your daily routines of sleeping, eating, working, playing, etc.

Maintenance Level

How can you calculate your *Maintenance Level?* Obviously any method you use will be only an approximation because of the host of variables which include body weight, personality type, enthusiasm for each day's activities, occupation, weather conditions, etc. However if individuals move about rather slowly or only when absolutely necessary, hold down sedentary desk jobs which are not stressful and watch television for recreation, they will probably obtain a quite accurate caloric *Maintencance Level* by multiplying their body weight in pounds by 12 calories. On that basis a 100 pound person would need approximately 1200 calories daily to maintain body weight with no significant gain or loss. However, if this individual were hyperactive and performing relatively hard physical labor which involved a fair amount of stress, 25 calories per pound might be required to maintain body weight without significant gain or loss. This person's *Maintenance Level* would be 2500 calories (100 pounds × 25 calories).

Here is some advice on how to decide what your level of activity might be and whether you should multiply your weight in pounds by 12 calories, 14 calories, 16 calories, or some higher figure up to 25 calories in calculating your approximate caloric *Maintenance Level*.

1. Is your only significant exercise getting to and from a non-stressful desk job? Do you lie down to watch television? Do you move about only when absolutely necessary? If this is your situation, multiply your weight in pounds by 12 to arrive at the approximate number of calories you will burn in 24 hours, your caloric *Maintenance Level*.

2. Do you have a relatively sedentary occupation or do only light housework? Do you prefer a passive rather than an active role in entertainment? Do you think you exercise less than most of your friends? If this profile fits your situation, multiply your weight in pounds by 14 to arrive at your caloric *Maintenance Level*.

3. If you consider yourself an average individual who is neither sedentary nor hyperactive but one who makes no special effort to exercise or get things accomplished quickly, multiply your weight in pounds by 16 to arrive at a reasonable estimate of your caloric maintenance requirements for each 24-hour day, your caloric *Maintenance Level*.

4. If you are quite active, if you tend to stand when you could sit, if you exercise for social or health reasons several times a week and if you are quite active in the workplace, multiply your weight in pounds by 18 to approximate your caloric maintenance requirement for a 24-hour day.

5. If you consider yourself hyperactive, if you pace the floor, if you often walk instead of riding, if you frequently use stairways in preference to elevators, if your occupation involves hard physical labor or if you exercise almost daily for health reasons,

you should probably multiply your weight in pounds by 20 in order to find your approximate *Maintenance Level.*

6. Of course if you happen to be extremely hyperactive and tense or perform hard physical labor in difficult weather conditions, you might need to multiply your weight in pounds by as much as 25 or more to find your true caloric *Maintenance Level.*

The following table can serve as a guide to calculating an approximate *Maintenance Level* for people of different weights, lifestyles and temperaments.

TABLE IV-1

Weight	Life-Style	Caloric Maintenance Level
100 lbs	Sedentary and Relaxed	1200 (12 cal/lb)
100 lbs	Hyperactive and Tense	2000 (20 cal/lb)
115 lbs	Sedentary and Relaxed	1380 (12 cal/lb)
115 lbs	Hyperactive and Tense	2300 (20 cal/lb)
130 lbs	Sedentary and Relaxed	1560 (12 cal/lb)
130 lbs	Hyperactive and Tense	2600 (20 cal/lb)
150 lbs	Sedentary and Relaxed	1800 (12 cal/lb)
150 lbs	Hyperactive and Tense	3000 (20 cal/lb)
170 lbs	Sedentary and Relaxed	2040 (12 cal/lb)
170 lbs	Hyperactive and Tense	3400 (20 cal/lb)
200 lbs	Sedentary and Relaxed	2400 (12 cal/lb)
200 lbs	Hyperactive and Tense	4000 (20 cal/lb)
250 lbs	Sedentary and Relaxed	3000 (12 cal/lb)
275 lbs	Sedentary and Relaxed	3300 (12 cal/lb)
300 lbs	Sedentary and Relaxed	3600 (12 cal/lb)
325 lbs	Sedentary and Relaxed	3900 (12 cal/lb)
350 lbs	Sedentary and Relaxed	4200 (12 cal/lb)

To summarize we may state that it has been estimated that a person with a sedentary and relaxed life-style will utilize about 12 calories per pound per day, and one who is hyperactive and tense will burn about 20 calories per pound per day.

From these data, one can estimate an approximate caloric *"Maintenance Level"* and calculate the number of calories which would be allowed daily if they chose to lose one pound of body fat (3500 calories) per week or two pounds per week (7000 calories).

Let us take, for example, a 130-pound individual who is neither sedentary and relaxed (12 cal/lb per day) nor hyperactive and tense (20 cal/lb per day). We might choose 15 cal/lb/day or 1950 calories per day as a fair approximation of that person's caloric *"Maintenance Level"*. If that person is going to lose one pound of body fat per week (3500 calories), the daily caloric intake must be cut by 500 calories for each of the seven days of the week. This means that instead of being allowed 1950 calories per day, only 1450 will be allowed. If this individual wishes to lose two pounds of fat (7000 calories), the daily intake must be cut to 950 calories or a decrease of 1000 calories per day, and that severe restriction might prove extremely difficult to continue for any protracted period of time.

Exercise, any increase in physical activity, will help you lose weight, but the extent to which it can augment the effects of a low-calorie diet can perhaps be best illustrated by a discussion of rapid walking, a physical activity we all understand and one in which most of us can participate. If you were a 140-pound person and were to walk extremely rapidly for 5 miles (13 min/mile), it would take you a little more than an hour and you would burn about 500 calories above your *Maintenance Level*. If you performed this rapid walking exercise (5 miles each day) for seven days, you would burn (500 cal × 7) 3500 excess calories or the equivalent of one pound of body fat. Once you completely understand these mathematics of weight loss, you should be better prepared to deal with unreasonable expectations engendered by many weight loss programs. Exercise is wonderful for your cardiovascular system (heart and blood vessels), but it cannot compete in effectiveness with the avoidance of rich foods in the weight-loss sweepstakes. The wisdom of avoiding the 1000 calorie ice cream sundae, which is the equivalent of two extremely rapid 5-mile walks, should now be more apparent to one intent on losing excess pounds of fat.

If you wish to use exercise as an aid to weight loss or as adjunct treatment for coronary heart disease, diabetes, incipient senile changes, etc., you may wish to know how many calories are utilized over and beyond those needed to maintain your body weight. In other words, how many calories are burned per hour above your *Maintenance Level* during a specific activity or exercise. Table IV-2 will serve as a guide.

TABLE IV-2

APPROXIMATE NUMBER OF *CALORIES* BURNED
PER HOUR ABOVE *MAINTENANCE LEVEL*

Activity	Weight 100 lbs calories burned per hour above M.L.	Weight 150 lbs calories burned per hour above M.L.	Weight 200 lbs. calories burned per hour above M.L.
Bowling	100	150	200
Walking (3 MPH)	100	150	200
Bicycling (5.5 MPH)	150	200	300
Golf (carry or drag clubs)	150	200	300
Walking (4 MPH)	200	300	400
Tennis	200	300	400
Bicycling (10 MPH)	250	400	500
Aerobic & Square Dancing	250	400	500
Swimming (Breaststroke)	250	400	500
Handball & Squash	300	500	650
Raquetball	300	500	650
Jogging (11 minutes/ mile)	300	500	650
Swimming (Crawl)	300	500	650
Skiing (Downhill)	300	500	650
Skiing (Cross-Country)	350	550	750
Running (8 minutes/ mile)	500	750	1000

Mark Twain said, "When I feel like exercising, I lie down until I get over the idea." That is very funny and certainly very entertaining, but it would be poor advice and in practice would tend to hasten our demise. This great humorist also said, "It is easy to stop smoking, I've done it a hundred times." That facetious remark emphasizes the fact that changing one's habits is extremely difficult. Of course it isn't easy to stop smoking, excessive drinking or overeating for any prolonged period of time. But these are keys to weight loss and good health.

Exercise daily, eat as much as you wish from the *Food Lists*, eat as often as you desire; but if you intend to lose weight, keep your caloric intake *below* your *Maintenance Level* by choosing the lower-calorie foods.

There is always some suffering involved in losing pound after pound of body fat, and many cannot force themselves to suffer for long periods of time unless there is no alternative. Only when they are faced with loss of promotion, loss of job security or loss of life from one of the degenerative diseases can they bring themselves to seriously consider weight loss. So they spend their time and energies looking for the easy solution, the quick "fix". They are forever "fad" dieting and never happy. They experience temporary successes followed by dismal failures.

They may decide, for example, to lose 10 pounds per week for four weeks and then revert to their old life-styles. Do they ever examine the mathematics of this sort of regimen? Of course they don't or they would immediately see the dangers and impracticalities involved. How could one lose 10 pounds of fat (10 × 3500 calories) or 35,000 calories in one week? Let us assume, for example, that this individual weighs 190 pounds, is working daily, and is moderately active (utilizing about 15 cal/lb/day). The caloric *"Maintenance Level"* would be 15 cal × 190 lbs or 2850 calories per day, or 19,950 calories per week. If this person ingested nothing but water (no calories) for one week (absolutely no food) and continued working daily and engaging in other ordinary activities, the weight loss would amount to slightly less than 6 pounds of body fat. To lose the additional 4 pounds by exercise to make the total body fat loss 10 pounds for the week, rapid walking (15 minutes/mile) could be chosen and this activity could burn approximately 100 additional calories per mile above the maintenance level. To lose the additional 4 pounds of body fat (14,000 calories) would require this individual to walk 140 miles. That amounts to 20 miles per day for each of the seven days to reach the goal. Does this sound like a reasonable program?

Let us be more realistic. Let us suppose that our 190-pound person wishes to lose 2 pounds of body fat per week, and let us assume that this individual is working daily and is moderately active (15 cal/lb/day) which means a caloric *Maintenance Level* of 2850 calories per day. The goal is a loss of two pounds of body fat, 7,000 calories, per week or 1,000 calories per day. Therefore this person could consume 1850 calories per day and lose the two pounds of body fat in a week. There are however other alternatives. Exercise could accomplish the two-pound weight loss. This person could continue to eat the 2800 calorie *Maintenance Level* diet and begin an exercise program of rapid walking (15 minutes per mile), but this would involve ten miles per day for each of the seven days of the week. Or calorie-cutting could be combined with exercise, a more sensible solution to the problem.

The foregoing information and examples should convince us that loss of body fat is much more dependent on the ingestion of low-calorie, high-fiber foods than on exercise. May I repeat? Exercise will burn calories and exercise is wonderful for your heart, lungs and arteries, but exercise without calorie-cutting can be a very time-consuming and difficult method of attaining weight loss. Correct nutrition combined with a daily, 30-minute, fairly strenuous exercise program will not only prevent obesity, but will cause loss of any excess pounds.

Summary

Keep in mind the fact that animals which forage in the wilds for food do not become too fat. These animals are expending energy and eating natural unrefined foods. In other words they are on a forced exercise program and an unrefined diet.

When one sees an obese animal, the sad plight of the poor beast is usually caused by an owner who is promoting under-

exercising with over-feeding of refined foods. When one sees
an obese human, the same factors are undoubtedly operating,
too little exercise and a preference for refined foods (especially
sugar, white rice, white flour and beer or ale).

Prevention of Obesity

1. The *Correct Nutrition* regimen detailed in Chapter II,
   which allows *no* refined carbohydrates (especially sugar,
   white rice, white flour and beer) and which stresses the
   consumption of large quantities of fresh, raw or steamed
   vegetables and fresh, raw fruit, will prevent obesity when
   coupled to the *Exercise Program* outlined in Chapter III.
2. The *Exercise Program* includes a rapid (thirty-minute),
   two mile walk daily, seven days a week.

Treatment of Obesity

1. Same as listed above under *Prevention of Obesity.*

Cure of Obesity

1. Same as listed above under *Prevention of Obesity.*

CHAPTER V

Arteriosclerosis
(Hardening of the Arteries)

Arteriosclerosis has frequently been referred to as "hardening of the arteries". It is a degenerative disease with thickening of blood vessel walls, often accompanied by calcification. In the minds of many people, it is associated mainly with old age and senility.

In this discussion, we shall deal primarily with a form of arteriosclerosis that is called atherosclerosis because of the formation of atherosclerotic plaque in the walls of arteries. This plaque may narrow or completely clog the lumen of an artery resulting in decreased blood flow or total stoppage.

Atherosclerosis is actually a degenerative disease of arterial walls that often begins in infancy. Whether it fails to develop significantly or progresses to cause disabling diseases depends mainly on the individual's diet. A correct nutrition and exercise program can not only prevent atherosclerosis but can also cause regression and cure even after it has been long established. In populations where unprocessed, natural plant foods form the major portion of the diet and in vegetarians the incidence of this affliction is low and the extent of its progression is diminished in those affected.

Atherosclerosis is the major cause of death in the United States today, and as early as 1965 it was accounting for more than 44% of deaths from all causes. Most atherosclerotic deaths come from atherosclerotic coronary heart disease and atherosclerotic cerebrovascular disease.

When atherosclerosis affects the arteries nourishing the heart, the patient becomes a candidate for angina, myocardial infarctions and "sudden death". When it blocks arteries nourishing the brain, cerebral thrombosis and "stroke" may occur and senile changes are common sequelae. Damage to the renal arteries supplying the kidneys may lead to hypertension and even kidney failure. Plaque formation in the abdominal aorta may lead to aortic aneurysm. When the arterial channels supplying blood to the legs and feet become increasingly narrowed, the patient may develop "intermittent claudication" (leg pain on walking short distances) with progression to cold, pulseless feet and necrotic ulcers with gangrene, often requiring amputation. And that is only an incomplete atherosclerosis disability list.

But atherosclerosis is preventable with correct nutrition and regular exercise. This should be the treatment of choice, even after it has become quite far advanced, for the only other effective treatments are palliative surgery such as arterial bypass and amputation.

See Chapter VI and VII for a more detailed discussion of the effects of atherosclerosis on the heart and brain.

Aortic Aneurysm

The term aneurysm refers to a weakening of the wall of an artery, usually caused by atherosclerotic disease, which results in a ballooning out and thinning of the arterial wall with the attendant danger of bursting or rupture, causing sudden, often fatal internal hemorrhage.

"Aortic aneurysms" are those involving the aorta, the largest blood vessel in the body. The most frequent location for one of these aneurysms is near the terminus of the aorta, as it lies on the vertebral column deep in the abdomen at about the level of the umbilicus or belly button. This aneurysm can often be easily felt as a large pulsating mass deep in the abdomen, and it is now possible to repair many of them surgically if they are recognized before they burst and cause fatal internal hemorrhage.

These aneurysms are caused by atherosclerosis, that degenerative disease which plagues the populations of the United States and Europe. If we could all change to a low-sugar, low-fat, high-fiber diet, "aortic aneurysm", a not infrequent cause of death, would become almost a thing of the past. It would almost disappear as a disease entity.

Diabetics are especially liable to develop these aneurysms, because atherosclerosis seems to progress much more rapidly in the presence of this disease. However, atherosclerosis is progressing constantly and relentlessly in all of us as long as we continue on the "Western" diet of high-sugar, high-fat, and low-fiber, and persist in our sedentary life-style.

The answer to the problem of prevention lies in the low-sugar, low-fat, high-fiber nutrition regimen detailed in Chapter II, combined with a regular, judiciously-organized exercise program.

Cardiac Arrhythmias

If we ever have the occasion to deal with the term, "cardiac arrhythmia", we should understand that it simply means that the heart is beating too fast, too slowly, or not regularly. These irregularities in rate, rhythm or both usually require evaluation by your physician, but they are not always serious or indicators of significant disease. Indeed, the heart may beat very rapidly (over 90 beats per minute) because of poor physical conditioning, emotional upset or relatively strenuous exertion. The heart rate may be very slow (40 to 50 beats per minute) in athletes in the "pink" of condition, because their hearts are so efficient that it takes fewer contractions to supply the body needs. So, rapid heart beats may simply indicate the need for a regular, well-constructed exercise program; and good physical condition may account for some of the slower rates. There are many other causes of arrhythmias including various kinds of heart damage, medications, and common chemicals, such as caffeine. Only your physician can advise you as to the correct course of action if you discover an irregularity, but each of us should be cognizant of a few of these basic facts. Irregular heart beat, even the not uncommon "skipped beat", indicates that something is amiss in the conduction system of the heart and the individual should be checked by a physician. The electrical impulses must pass through the heart's specialized conduction system and the main mass of heart muscle in an orderly manner; otherwise, irregular beats, an arrhythmia, may result. This is often reflected in a correspondingly irregular pulse rate at the wrist.

You should learn how to count your pulse so that you will be able to note irregularities in rhythm, or sudden marked changes in rate, should any occur. These observations, when told to your doctor, may enable the physician to make quickly a more precise assessment of the seriousness of the problem when confronted with it.

The things you eat and drink, the amount of regular physical exercise you get and the medications or drugs (alcohol, caffeine, etc.) you ingest may have a great deal to do with any "cardiac arrhythmias", sometimes directly and sometimes indirectly.

We have mentioned the relatively rapid heart rate of the person in poor physical condition and the irregularities that can be caused by caffeine, but of far greater significance are irregularities caused by damage to the conduction system of the heart by atherosclerotic coronary heart disease. Most of us can improve our physical condition quite easily. We can avoid caffeine (coffee, tea, chocolate, and many of the caffeine-containing soft drinks), but did you know that you could cure, by causing improved blood supply, some of the cardiac irregularities that are due to atherosclerotic coronary heart disease, the major cause of many of the most dangerous "cardiac arrhythmias"? To cure or to be almost certain of preventing a worsening of atherosclerotic coronary heart disease, one must change his or her life-style. Medications and surgical procedures are palliative, not curative, and are often not the answer. The patient must combine correct nutrition with a carefully supervised exercise program, otherwise the atherosclerotic plaque continues to build up and clog the arteries to the heart, including those to the specialized muscle of the heart's electrical conduction system. When the conduction system is damaged by poor blood supply, arrhythmias result.

Summary

Atherosclerosis as previously stated is a degenerative disease of the arteries that is responsible for the aortic aneurysms and many of the cardiac arrhythmias discussed in this chapter. It is also the major cause of coronary heart disease and "stroke" which are the subjects of subsequent chapters.

There is much controversy regarding the cause of atherosclerosis but there are certain studies which provide some valuable clues. Those populations subsisting on mainly coarse, natural, unrefined foods and the true vegetarians in our "Western" society tend to show little evidence of atherosclerotic disease. But we in the developed nations on the high-sugar, "Western" diet may begin to show evidence of atherosclerotic arterial damage in early childhood and the disease then progresses in severity throughout our lives causing many thousands of us to die every year of aneurysms, coronary heart disease, "stroke," etc. You may find it also quite interesting that experimental animals, such as monkeys will rapidly develop atherosclerosis on a diet high in refined sugar and will almost as rapidly be cured of their disease by changing their diet to one of coarse, natural unrefined foods. The same results are being obtained in humans but the studies are difficult to control and span long time periods. These anecdotes should cause you to think seriously about the advisability of remaining on the "Western" diet that is so high in refined sugar.

Prevention of Atherosclerosis

1. The *Correct Nutrition* regimen detailed in Chapter II, which allows *no* refined carbohydrates (especially sugar, white rice, white flour and beer) and which stresses the consumption of large quantities of fresh, raw or steamed vegetables and fresh, raw fruit, can prevent atherosclerosis and actually cause it to regress, provided that it is coupled to the *Exercise Program* outlined in Chapter III.
2. The *Exercise Program* includes a rapid (thirty-minute), two mile walk *daily,* seven days a week.

Treatment of Atherosclerosis

1. Same *Correct Nutrition* regimen and *Exercise Program* as
   listed above under *Prevention of Atherosclerosis* except
   that the rapid (thirty-minute), two-mile walks should be
   twice daily, seven days a week.

Cure of Atherosclerosis

1. Same as listed above under *Treatment of Atherosclerosis*.

CHAPTER VI

Coronary or Ischemic Heart Disease

The term coronary or ischemic heart disease implies that there is diminished blood flow to the heart muscle resulting in a damaged heart. By far the most common cause of the ischemia (diminished blood supply) is atherosclerosis. The heart muscle is nourished by oxygen-rich blood flowing through the coronary arteries in the heart walls. When these vessels become partially filled with atherosclerotic plaque, ischemia occurs in heart muscle and the condition may be designated either coronary heart disease, ischemic heart disease, arteriosclerotic heart disease or atherosclerotic coronary heart disease.

A National Health Survey has indicated that there are about 5 million Americans known to have ischemic heart disease, and there are many millions more with atherosclerotic disease in their coronary arteries that is daily progressing in severity, but may not have yet reached the stage of actually damaging heart muscle. Many of these individuals may be in greater danger than those who recognize that they have damaged hearts, because the former may be doing nothing in the realms of prevention or cure. We know that atherosclerotic disease may begin in infancy and often continues to build-up throughout life at various rates among different individuals depending mainly on lifestyle, such as type of diet, amount of cigarette smoking and the level of physical activity.

Heart disease is the leading cause of death in the United States today for both men and women, and atherosclerotic coronary heart disease, with its catastrophic complications of myocardial infarction and "sudden death", is the major contributor to this statistic.

It is now possible to indentify practically all persons at risk of developing ischemic heart disease and a list of these "risk factors" includes the following:

1. "Western" Diet—This diet is high in sugars, fats, and processed and packaged foods. It is the major cause of atherosclerotic heart disease.

2. Lack of Regular, Relatively Strenuous Exercise.

3. Obestiy—This is a common consequence of the "Western" diet.

4. Cigarette Smoking—This seems to accelerate the atherosclerotic disease.

5. Hypertension—High blood pressure increases the risk of coronary heart disease by accelerating the atherosclerotic process.

6. Hyperlipidemia—This is adversely influenced by the "Western " diet.

7. Diabetes Mellitus—Diabetes seems to accelerate the atherosclerotic arterial changes.

8. Family History—There are probably genetic factors as well as environmental influences at work in atherosclerotic arterial disease, and one is definitely at increased risk of atherosclerotic disease if it has affected family members or other blood relatives.

9. Age—The amount of atherosclerotic arterial damage increases directly with increased age.

Discussion of Risk Factors

1. "Western" Diet—Why is the "Western" diet a risk factor in ischemic heart disease? Simply put, the high-sugar, high-fat, low-fiber diet is the major cause of atherosclerosis, which is the major cause of ischemic heart disease. The atherosclerotic plaque narrows the vascular channels and impedes the blood flow through the coronary arteries. This leads to myocardial infarctions, cardiac arrhythmias and "sudden death".

2. Lack of Regular, Relatively Strenuous Exercise—We must have a regular exercise program if we are to avoid atheroscle-

rosis. Two examples can illustrate quite well the benefit of exercise. It was found that Postal Service Letter-Carriers who walked their mail routes day after day and year after year had a much lower incidence of coronary heart disease than did their peers who had sedentary desk jobs back at the post office. Another study showed that the drivers of double-decker London buses had a higher rate of coronary heart disease than did the ticket-collectors who rode at the back of the bus. These persons were constantly on their feet and frequently climbed the steep narrow stairways to the top deck to collect fares, thus getting far more exercise than the drivers. Lack of regular physical exercise is a most important risk factor.

3. Obesity—The Framingham study has shown a higher incidence of angina (chest pain on exertion) and "sudden death" from ischemic heart disease in men between 45 and 62 years of age whose weights were 20% or more above the "norm" or whose weights had increased significantly after age 25.

4. Cigarette Smoking—The death rate for cigarette smokers increases in proportion to the number of cigarettes smoked. If you are addicted to cigarettes, you are at tremendously increased risk of "sudden death" due to atherosclerotic heart disease, in part because your chances of "sudden death" increase dramatically when other risk factors combine with the effects of smoking cigarettes; and cigarette smokers who die of unrelated causes (auto accidents, etc.) are found at autopsy to have more atherosclerosis than non-smokers.

If there is one thing you can do, in addition to correct nutrition and regular physical exercise, that will reduce your risk of "sudden death" or becoming incapacitated by coronary heart disease, it is *Stop Smoking Cigarettes.*

5. Hypertension—In the Framingham Study, men in the age group 45 to 62 who had high blood pressure exceeding 165/95 had 5 times the rate of coronary heart disease when compared with the incidence in those with blood pressure below 140/90. This and other studies indicate quite clearly that hypertension increases dramatically the danger of coronary heart disease and "sudden death". The moral here seems to be to have your blood pressure checked at least annually and avail yourself of these correct nutrition and exercise programs to either maintain your pressure at a normal level or to serve as adjuct treatment should

it become elevated or remain elevated despite correct nutrition and exercise.

6. Hyperlipidemia—This "risk factor" raises very complicated issues, but the majority of cases can be controlled by the correct nutrition and exercise programs. Annual testing of the cholesterol and triglyceride levels in the blood usually serve as quite reliable guides to the the effectiveness of these programs in correcting and controlling the blood lipid levels. Despite what your physician may tell you, if your "cholesterol" is over 150 or your "triglycerides" are over 100, you may quite probably be building atheromatous plaque in your arterial walls. This plaque tends to narrow and block the blood channels, obstructing the free flow of blood. If this happens in your coronary arteries, it may lead to "sudden death" or other less major disasters.

7. Diabetes Mellitus—If you have a family history of sugar diabetes (relatives with diabetes), you are much more at risk than are those with negative family histories, both for developing diabetes yourself and for having accelerated atherosclerotic arterial disease with coronary heart disease. Therefore, any diabetic or anyone with a family history of diabetes should shun the "Western" diet and the sedentary life-style.

8. Family History—If members of your family (blood relatives such as parents, grandparents, aunts, uncles, brothers or sisters) have had angina pectoris (a type of chest pain on exertion) or "sudden death" due to coronary heart disease, statistics show that you are at greater risk than the general population. Whether this is genetic or environmental is moot or debatable, but prevention of this increased risk will depend on decreasing other risk factors, with special attention to correct nutrition, regular physical exercise, and avoiding cigarette smoking.

9. Age—Age is obviously a risk factor for "sudden death" from coronary heart disease. Atherosclerotic disease of the arterial walls causes more and more clogging of the blood channels as the years pass by. The longer we stay on the "Western" diet and embrace a sedentary existence, the more we develop plaque and the more we block the free flow of blood to the heart and other vital organs. However, even though this atherosclerotic process may progress in severity for years, it can be halted and even made to regress by changing to a specific, correct nutrition regi-

men, joined to a judiciously chosen, regular exercise program. It should be no suprise that death from atherosclerotic coronary heart disease is the leading cause of death in the Western world (United States and Europe), that the incidence of this dread affliction tends to increase with age and that only an educated change in life-style (nutrition and physical activity) can alter the situation significantly.

After studying the risk factors associated with atherosclerotic ischemic heart disease, one may reasonably conclude that many of these risk factors can be avoided with little suffering, except for the "withdrawal pains" associated with the cure of "addictions" such as sugar, fats and cigarettes. Alcohol might also present a problem. Alcohol intake should be held to a "reasonable level". In this instance "reasonable" is difficult to define. For the alcoholic, it is a "zero" level of consumption. For most of us, it is a "low" level. Alcohol adds calories but nothing else of significant value, thus contributing nothing to health but much to weight gain and obesity.

We suffer the terrible anxieties and intense chest pains of angina pectoris, we clutter the hospital intensive care units with cases of myocardial infarction, we submit to coronary bypass surgery, and we die of atheromatous coronary heart disease. Why does this happen? It is simply that we eat too much and too many of the wrong foods, improperly cook or prepare many foods and lead too sedentary a life-style (too little regular, judicious physical exercise).

When are we going to realize that in the vast majority of these cases of atherosclerotic heart disease, we don't need potentially dangerous medications and extremely hazardous heart surgery to lead a life free of the complications of atherosclerotic disease with the severe chest pains, the expensive, miserable, time-consuming stays in hospital intensive care units, and the fear of "sudden death"? The sensible answer lies in prevention, not in prescription drugs and major surgery. The sensible answer is correct nutrition and a regular, carefully selected and designed exercise program.

Correct nutrition, coupled with a well-designed exercise program, can not only *prevent* atherosclerotic coronary heart disease, but it can *cure* it in many instances. Atheromatous plaques, which narrow the arterial blood channels and impede blood flow to the heart muscle, can be caused by poor nutrition. However, a correct nutrition regimen combined with a regular exercise program can halt the growth or accumulation of plaque and actually cause regression of the disease process with increased blood flow. Prescription drugs and coronary bypass surgery do not *cure* atherosclerotic heart disease. They are palliative procedures designed to provide temporary relief for immediate problems. Without correct nutrition and exercise programs following bypass surgery, coronary arteries will continue to fill with plaque and the new bypass vessels will also succumb to the atherosclerotic narrowing and clogging and will become non-functional and useless.

If one wishes to avoid angina pectoris, coronary occlusion, myocardial infarction or "sudden death", or if one wishes to effect regression or permanent cure of atherosclerotic coronary heart disease, the best treatment is not medicine or open-heart surgery but a correct nutrition regimen and exercise program. This involves a change in life-style, but it has so much more to offer than medicine or surgery. The prospect of cure should be much more palatable than the palliative effects of sometimes dangerous drugs or the often only temporarily beneficial results of arterial bypass with open-heart surgery.

Summary

It is certainly of interest to note that the incidence of coronary or ischemic heart disease is very low among energetic populations subsisting on a diet of mainly coarse, unrefined carbohydrates and is likewise very low in the Eskimoes living primitively on a diet high in protein and fat. However, when either of these groups of people is introduced to the high-sugar, "Western" diet, they begin to develop atherosclerosis, which after about thirty years will cause them to begin dying of coronary or ischemic heart disease, an affliction to which they were formerly seemingly immune. Just as coronary disease has become epidemic in our "Western" populations on a high-sugar, low-fiber diet, so does it become epidemic in any group of people who join us in consuming large amounts of refined carbo-hydrates *(especially refined sugar).*

If our health care resources are limited, perhaps we should allocate more to education of the public on the best methods of preventing, treating and curing this dreadful affliction rather than on CPR (cardiopulmonary resuscitation) training and ICUs (intensive care units) which are directed not at prevention but more toward handling the patients after they have been stricken by this perilous disease.

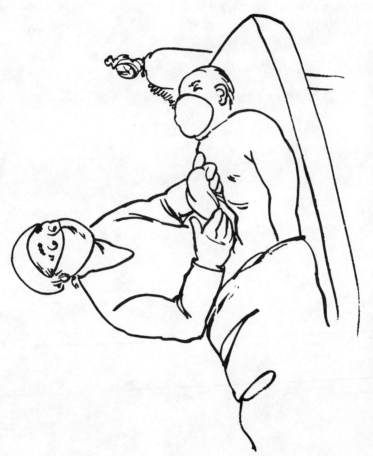

ILLUSTRATION VI-1

Prevention of Coronary or Ischemic Heart Disease

1. The *Correct Nutrition* regimen detailed in Chapter II, which allows *no* refined carbohydrates (especially sugar, white rice, white flour and beer) and which stresses the consumption of large quantities of fresh, raw or steamed vegetables and fresh, raw fruit, can prevent coronary heart disease if coupled with an *Exercise Program* which includes a rapid (thirty-minute), two-mile walk *daily*, seven days a week.

Treatment of Coronary or Ischemic Heart Disease

1. The *Correct Nutrition* regimen as listed above for *Prevention of Coronary or Ischemic Heart Disease.*
2. An *Exercise Program* designed by your physician for your unique situation that will result ultimately in *two*, rapid (thirty-minute), two mile walks *daily*, seven days a week.

Cure of Coronary or Ischemic Heart Disease

1. Same *Correct Nutrition* regimen as noted above for *Prevention of Coronary or Ischemic Heart Disease.*
2. Same *Exercise Program* as listed under *Treatment of Coronary or Ischemic Heart Disease* with the reminder that it must be designed and monitored by your physician.

CHAPTER VII

Atherosclerotic Cerebrovascular Disease, Stroke and Senility

Atherosclerotic cerebrovascular disease is a degenerative disease involving a thickening of the walls of arteries supplying blood to the brain. The narrowing of the vascular channels tends to slow and obstruct the flow of blood. This invites intravascular thrombosis or clotting of blood which may then occlude a narrowed artery completely. The diminished or totally abolished blood supply then causes damage or death of the brain tissue which depends upon that artery for nourishment.

Over 80% of "paralytic strokes" are the direct result of this narrowing of the arterial blood channels caused by atherosclerotic thickening and plaque formation in the vessel walls. The inflamed surfaces of atherosclerotic plaque encourage the formation of the blood clots or thrombi, which may then cause complete obstruction to blood flow. Any resulting loss of sensation or any paralysis would be called a "stroke" or cerebral thrombosis or cerebrovascular accident.

Multiple small "strokes" may occur intermittently over long periods of time and eventually culminate in such wide-spread brain damage that the resulting mental deterioration may become very similar to that seen in Alzheimer's disease and senile dementia. The insidious occurrence of the first small "strokes" with perhaps very minor physical or mental disabilities may pass virtually unnoticed or be considered unremarkable by the family. When less subtle changes occur such as memory lapses, incontinence of urine and physical incapacities, they are often viewed as the inevitable accompaniments of old age or in a younger person as an example of early aging. Major "strokes", with marked changes in sensation, paralysis of muscles on one side of the body and freqently an inability to speak (expressive aphasia) are easily recognized by almost anyone.

Atherosclerosis of the cerebral vessels with resulting cerebral thrombosis and "stroke" have never been absolutely proven to be diet related, but it is certainly not unreasonable to assume that if diet is related to atherosclerosis in the other arteries of the body, it is quite probably related to those nourishing the brain.

Certainly both prevention and treatment of cerebrovascular disease should begin with correct nutrition and the institution of an exercise program specifically tailored to the unique needs of each individual. Our nursing homes and retirement homes are filled with people who badly need the benefits of both the preventative and the treatment aspects of these dietary and exercise programs to prevent or slow the onset of senility.

Summary

In Chapter V we learned that atherosclerosis could be prevented, treated and in many cases even cured by *Correct Nutrition* and *exercise.* In Chapter VI we found that the atherosclerotic damage to the arteries supplying the heart could be prevented and even made to regress. In this chapter we have learned how this degenerative disease, assaulting the arteries of the brain, can cause "strokes" and senility, and we will find that prevention and treatment will be the same as for atherosclerosis elsewhere, for it involves attacking the atherosclerotic disease in the same manner wherever it may occur.

**Prevention of Atherosclerotic
Cerebrovascular Disease,
Strokes and Senility**

1. The *Correct Nutrition* regimen detailed in Chapter II,

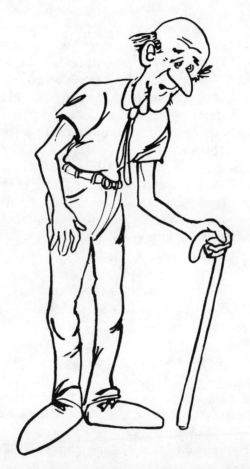

TOOTHLESS, SENILE, RHEUMATIC!!
AND ALL PREVENTABLE!!

ILLUSTRATION VII-1

which allows *no* refined carbohydrates (especially sugar, white rice and white flour) and which stresses the consumption of large quantities of fresh, raw or steamed vegetables and fresh, raw fruit, can prevent atherosclerotic disease of the blood vessels supplying the brain and thus diminish the likelihood of "strokes" and senile changes, especially when combined with an *Exercise Program* such as that detailed in Chapter III.

Treatment of Atherosclerotic Cerebrovascular Disease

1. Same *Correct Nutrition* regimen as listed above under *Prevention of Atherosclerotic Cerebrovascular Disease.*
2. An *Exercise Program* designed by the patient's physician that is appropriate for that patient's unique situation and physical condition. This program should consist of *two* exercise periods *daily,* seven days a week. Each exercise period should include a thirty-minute walk, if and when the patient can tolerate safely this much activity. The rapidity and length of the walks may be gradually increased to whatever speed and distance can subsequently be safely and reasonably attained in the thirty-minute periods.

Cure of Atherosclerotic Cerebrovascular Disease

1. The *Correct Nutrition* regimen as detailed in Chapter II, which allows *absolutely no* refined carbohydrates (especially sugar, white rice and white flour and *absolutely no* alcoholic drinks or cigarettes and which stresses the consumption of large quantities of fresh, raw or steamed vegetables and fresh, raw fruit, can cure many cases of atherosclerotic cerebrovascular disease if combined with an appropriate *Exercise Program.*
2. The *Exercise Program* should be the one detailed above under *Treatment of Cerebrovascular Disease* and must be physician approved.

CHAPTER VIII

Hypertension (High Blood Pressure)

"Hypertension" (high blood pressure) is a chronic disease, and a treatment program must be designed that is compatible with a lifelong commitment to therapy. If potentially toxic drugs are used, one must attempt to balance the possible harmful effects against the probable good. This often creates a dilemma, and since medications frequently have different effects on different individuals, the physician may have to make extremely difficult and important decisions.

High blood pressure has been defined quite clearly by the actuarial studies compiled by insurance companies over many, many years. A systolic reading of 140 may be considered to be beyond the upper limit of normal. However, we appreciate the fact that the systolic value is of much less consequence than the diastolic and that many persons with a systolic pressure over 140, provided that their diastolic is less than 90, may be in absolutely no jeopardy related to their blood pressure. A diastolic blood pressure of 90 or above, however, is a danger signal that we cannot disregard or take lightly. The elevated diastolic reading (90 or higher), if found consistently, usually indicates increased vascular resistance, and a treatment program should be instituted at once.

In at least 90% of cases of hypertension, no cause can be found, and many of these patients exhibit no diagnostic signs and have no symptoms or complaints. However, one early symptom may be that of a dull, pounding headache in the back of the head which is often present on waking in the morning and which tends to wear off or disappear during the day.

Statistics from insurance companies show unequivocally that individuals with hypertension have, in general, a decreased life-expectancy. This makes it mandatory that we put forth concentrated efforts to get the many millions of hypertensives to at least be aware that they have high blood pressure and that it is a treatable problem. They should be made to realize that their life-expectancy can, in the vast majority of cases, be extended to a normal or very near normal life-span if early and continuous treatment is instituted and unrelentingly followed.

The safest, simplest and best beginning treatment for mild hypertensives is the nutrition regimen outlined in Chapter II (except that there should be no salt added to food) combined with a judiciously chosen regular exercise program that is uniquely designed for the individual. If these programs should fail to lower the blood pressure to normal levels (below 140/90) after three months, the physician will probably prescribe medication. If these medications are successful in lowering your blood pressure and maintaining it below 140/90, your doctor will then undoubtedly begin decreasing the dosages of the drugs until they may be no longer needed. At this point, you may maintain your normal blood pressure with your nutrition and exercise programs, but you will be well-advised to have your pressure monitored frequently and regularly to be certain that you continue to remain free of danger.

You should be aware that many prescription drugs may be hazardous to your health and to your general feeling of well-being, and they should be taken only under the careful guidance of your physician. Some of the possible side-effects of a list of prescription drugs for hypertension include arthritis, headache, nausea, impotence, tremor, hallucinations, depression, sedation, fatigue, potassium depletion, hyperglycemia, hyperuricemia, and a host of others. If the recommended nutrition regimen and exercise program can control your hypertension by bringing your blood pressure down and maintaining it within normal limits, or even lower the amount of medication needed to control it, you will have made your treatment program safer. Also, by changing your eating and exercise habits, you would be halting the progress of other degenerative diseases such as atherosclerotic coronary heart disease, cerebrovascular disease and many more.

Of course, it is much easier to take "pills" than to change one's life-style. It is also less time-consuming. But, is it worth the risk if it is not absolutely necessary?

Obviously there will always be patients who will need one or more relatively hazardous medications to control their disease. But keep in mind that a great many will need no medication at all, if they have the will and the moral fiber to change their life-style.

Summary

You should be made aware that many of us have proven that our patients' blood pressures can be controlled at normal levels by correct nutrition and exercise alone. Many others of our patients have had the dosages of their hypertension medications lowered markedly, simply by adding the adjunct treatment of correct nutrition and exercise to their treatment programs. They have thus put themselves at less risk of adverse reactions from potent and not infrequently hazardous medication.

Prevention of Hypertension
(High Blood Pressure)

1. We are certainly not advocating the following change in life-style as a panacea, but it will surely exert beneficial effects.
2. The *Correct Nutrition* regimen detailed in Chapter II, which allows *no* refined carbohydrates (especially sugar, white rice and white flour) and which stresses the consumption of large quantities of fresh, raw or steamed vegetables and fresh, raw fruit, when coupled to an *Exercise Program* will prevent many cases of hypertension from developing or progressing.

Treatment of Hypertension

1. The *Correct Nutrition* regimen detailed in Chapter II should be the first step in treatment.
2. The *Exercise Program*, designed by your physician, should be the second step in treatment.
3. Abolishing the use of salt in the kitchen and at the dining table *may* be a necessary third step in treatment (most of us should probably use less salt than we do).
4. Medication, prescribed by your physician, may be a necessary fourth step in treatment, but only in those cases where correct nutrition, exercise and reasonable salt restriction will not suffice.

Cure of Hypertension

1. Cure can be attained in many cases of mild hypertension for as long as the patient is willing to adhere to *Correct Nutrition* coupled with a suitable *Exercise Program*.
2. The above change in life-style will often make medication unnecessary. When medication is necessary, despite correct nutrition and exercise, the dosage will be smaller and consequently safer.

CHAPTER IX

Diabetes Mellitus

There are perhaps 200 million diabetics in the world, probably 4 million in the United States. This is obviously a very common disease, and it is extremely important to be aware of any possible preventative measures. The vascular complications alone create massive public health problems, and this malady is a major contributor to the vast numbers of persons dying every year from coronary heart disease and cerebral thrombosis or "stroke".

It has been estimated that nearly 50% of the 4 million diabetics in this country do not know they have the disease. This is true mainly because diabetes may smolder relatively silently for years, with the patient having no suspicion of the problem. However, during all the time the disease goes on undetected, and thus untreated, the patient's body is being ravaged. The damage to the coronary arteries supplying the heart make the diabetic prone to myocardial infarction and "sudden death". The blood vessels nourishing the brain undergo narrowing and clogging so that the incidence of "paralytic stroke" increases markedly. The damaged arteries supplying the kidneys cause kidney damage and anemia. The atherosclerosis in the blood vessels supplying the eyes may result in blurred vision, which often progresses to blindness. In fact, diabetes accounts for one-third of all the blindness in the United States. This generalized vascular damage also includes the arteries supplying the lower extremities and feet, and often results in ulceration and gangrene, especially in the elderly, so that amputation becomes a relatively common surgical procedure in older diabetics. One estimate indicates that amputation may be 150 times as common in diabetics as in non-diabetics.

In this discussion, we will concentrate on the "adult-onset" or "maturity-onset" type of diabetes. By this, we mean the form of the disease that has its beginning later in life, as distinguished from the insulin dependent "juvenile-onset" form of the disease which makes its appearance early.

The "mature onset" diabetic patient is usually overweight or obese and symptoms may be minimal or absent. Some of the signs which may alert the patient and bring him or her to a testing center or physician include pruritus (itching) of the genital region of the female, male impotence (inability to function sexually), nocturia (rising at night to urinate), ease of fatigue (abnormal tiredness), blurred vision, slow healing of minor trauma such as cuts and scratches, loss of sensation in the feet and hands and ulcer or gangrene of a toe or heel.

Of the 4 million diabetics in the United States, 50% do not know they have the disease, and since properly-treated diabetics generally do not develop many of the complications, it becomes extremely important to identify all persons harboring the disease and all who are at risk of developing it. Perhaps as many as 85% of "mature-onset" diabetics are grossly overweight or obese, so all overweight and obese individuals should be tested regularly by their physicians or by some diabetes testing center. At increased risk of being diabetic also are relatives of diabetics, for both genetics and environmental influences are factors in producing the disease. Also, inasmuch as the probability of developing diabetes increases markedly with age, the medical check-up of the elderly patient for this malady should be performed more regularly and frequently.

Treatment should begin with prevention, and prevention is often possible with the loss of the excess fat and attainment of a normal weight combined with a correct nutrition and exercise program. The patient who is diabetic must of course be in the care of a physician; but the nutrition regimen must be the one outlined in Chapter II, or one very similar; otherwise, the atherosclerotic damage to the blood vessels will continue, irrespective of any other treatment such as insulin or oral hypoglycemic drugs. Statistics show that over 50% of diabetics die of coronary heart disease. The degenerative processes may be slowed by drugs, but they will continue inexorably in the absence of correct nutrition and regular exercise, even more rapidly than they do in the non-diabetic. The danger of senile changes, paralytic strokes, and coronary heart disease with its dreaded complications of myocardial infarction and "sudden death", all of which are more frequent in diabetics, will continue to haunt those who ignore the constant worsening of the atherosclerotic blood vessel damage being caused by the disregard of correct nutrition and regular, daily, rather strenuous exercise (rapid walking for 30 minutes twice daily).

Summary

The results of several very interesting studies should be briefly mentioned before beginning a discussion of specifics of prevention and treatment of diabetes mellitus.

First, diabetes is on the increase as insurance company statistics have proven. However, this disease was always relatively uncommon until the refining of sugar and improved general economic conditions gave millions of people the opportunity to change their diets from one of coarse, natural, unrefined foods with low-sugar content to one high in refined sugar.

Second, let us begin with a question. How does the incidence of diabetes in rural China, India and Africa, where coarse, natural, unrefined carbohydrates form the mainstay of the diet, compare with the incidence of diabetes in those same races when they migrate to the cities or to countries where they become exposed to the high-sugar "Western" type diet? The answer is what we might at this point expect. The incidence of this disease, after a few decades, shoots upward and soon approaches that of the new culture.

Third, let us look at what happened when sugar was rationed in World War I and World War II. In both instances the mortality rate from diabetes plunged downward. After World War I the rate immediately shot upwards again. However, the discovery of antibiotics and the newer insulins combined with improved medical care have kept the mortality rate at a relatively low level since World War II and have allowed most diabetics to die of coronary heart disease rather than their diabetes specifically. You may recall that over 50% of diabetics now die of coronary heart disease.

Fourth, epidemiological research has shown conclusively that in populations where the consumption of refined sugar is high, the incidence of diabetes in high, and where the consumption of refined sugar is low, the incidence of diabetes is low.

Prevention of Diabetes Mellitus

1. The *Correct Nutrition* regimen detailed in Chapter II, which allows *no* refined carbohydrates (especially sugar, white rice, white flour and beer) and which stresses the consumption of large quantities of fresh, raw or steamed vegetables and fresh, raw fruit, can prevent diabetes and is the number one priority in preventive treatment.
2. The *Exercise Program* detailed in Chapter III which includes a rapid (thirty-minute), two-mile walk *daily,* seven days a week is the number two prevention priority.
3. Avoidance of excess weight and obesity is also of major importance.

Treatment of Diabetes Mellitus

1. The *Correct Nutrition* regimen detailed in Chapter II is the number one priority. You must quit stressing the pancreas with refined sugar. This regimen allows *no* refined carbohydrates (especially sugar, white rice and white flour) and no alcoholic drinks or sugared soft drinks and it stresses the consumption of large quantities of fresh, raw or steamed vegetables and fresh, raw fruit.
2. An *Exercise Program,* designed or approved by your physician, should include *two* (thirty-minute) walks *daily,* seven days a week. These walks should eventually become rapid (thirty-minute), two-mile walks and are the number two treatment priority.
3. Loss of excess weight or obesity is also essential.

4. Your physician will prescribe any needed medication such as insulin if necessary.

Cure of Diabetes Mellitus

1. The *Treatment of Diabetes Mellitus* outlined above will effect a cure, requiring no medication, in *many* cases for as long as the treatment program is strictly adhered to, for on this program the pancreas is not being continually stressed and damaged by refined sugars causing precipitous elevations in the blood sugar levels.

Hypoglycemia

The term "hypoglycemia" means low blood sugar, and there are many forms and diverse causes. The type of "hypoglycemia" here under discussion is the common "reactive functional hypoglycemia", which occurs almost without exception in patients who have emotional problems.

The maintenance of a constant level of glucose in the blood is absolutely essential to normal body function. The level of blood glucose at any time reflects a balance between two physiologic processes. One removes glucose from the blood to nourish the cells of the body such as those of the brain, liver and muscle or stores glucose in the liver and muscle as glycogen or in the adipose tissue as fat. The other process contributing to this physiological balance adds glucose to the blood by absorbing the products of digestion, forming glucose from non-glucose storage areas or mobilizing glycogen from storage depots.

The signs and symptoms of "hypoglycemia" include hunger, weakness, inward trembling, tachycardia (fast heart-rate) and sweating. The vast majority of cases can be prevented by a low-fat diet which stresses the avoidance of simple sugars and which substitutes in their place the natural and complex unrefined carbohydrates such as fresh fruits and vegetables, whole-grain products and legumes, all of which are more slowly digested. Such a diet is detailed in the nutrition regimen in Chapter II.

How does this diet tend to prevent both hyperglycemia (high blood sugar, as in diabetes) and hypoglycemia (low blood sugar)? When large amounts of glucose are quickly released into the blood stream in the process of digestion of sugars, hyperglycemia results, and the β or beta cells of the pancreas produce a surge of insulin to bring about utilization of this oversupply of glucose. The production of insulin by the pancreas then gradually slows, but it continues producing more insulin than needed for some time and this accounts for the hypoglycemic lows. However, our diet, low in sugar and high in natural foods (see Chapter II), causes slower release of the products of digestion, less stress on the pancreas and modification of both the hyperglycemic highs and the hypoglycemic lows. It should be apparent that this is the program to be used in the treatment of patients with hypoglycemia. Also, because it does not stress the insulin-forming pancreatic β or beta cells, it becomes the diet of choice of diabetics.

Prevention of Hypoglycemia

1. The *Correct Nutrition* regimen detailed in Chapter II, which allows *no* refined carbohydrates (especially sugar, white rice and white flour) and *no* alcoholic drinks and which stresses the consumption of large quantities of fresh, raw or steamed vegetables and fresh, raw fruit, can prevent low blood sugar levels or hypoglycemia, especially when coupled with the *Exercise Program* detailed in Chapter III.

Treatment of Hypoglycemia

1. Same as detailed above under *Prevention of Hypoglycemia.*

CHAPTER X

Peptic Ulcer

"Peptic ulcers" are commonly referred to by the lay public as "stomach ulcers", although actually probably 80% of them occur in the proximal portion of the duodenum (that part of the small intestine nearest the stomach). It has been estimated that 10% of all individuals will have a "peptic ulcer" at some period in their lifetime; however, some ulcers seem to be relatively silent or asymptomatic and thus may go undetected.

"Peptic ulcers" are a major cause of "indigestion", "gas", "bloating", "pain" and vague abdominal discomfort. They are most frequently found in the duodenum (duodenal ulcer), but often occur in the stomach (gastric ulcer) and with much less frequency elsewhere in the gastrointestinal tract.

Many theories have been propounded to explain the reason for the development of "peptic ulcer", but no single explanation can satisfactorily account for the occurrence of all of these lesions at the various sites at which they are found. "Peptic ulcers" may be produced experimentally by stress; and other psychological factors may play a definite role in the development of many, but these are, in the author's opinion, minor and secondary causes. Many of the more important generators of peptic ulceration are iatric. Chemical irritation of the stomach and intestine by proprietary medicines and prescription drugs are widely recognized as causative agents of gastritis (inflammation of the stomach lining) and of "peptic ulcer" as well. Surgical procedures involving the stomach and small intestines (even when carried out in an effort to cure "peptic ulcer" by excision) may actually create conditions causing peptic ulcers. However, the major cause of "peptic ulcer" is incorrect nutrition, which is often complicated by an accompanying obesity.

The suffering engendered by "peptic ulcer" is incalculable. As stated previously, 10% of the population will experience a "peptic ulcer" in their lifetime, and thousands will die in the United States every year as a result of "peptic ulcer" disease, many from massive hemorrhage and many others from perforation (bursting) and peritonitis. Millions of people live on baking soda, antacids and bland foods in an attempt to obtain relief from this frequently agonizing, often seriously incapacitating and sometimes fatal affliction. Major surgical procedures have been designed to cure this malady, but success has often been elusive and many sufferers have developed more serious problems after surgery than they had prior to the operation, including more "peptic ulcers".

Prevention of "peptic ulcer" can be accomplished safely and simply by a change in life-style. Strict adherence to correct nutrition is the answer. It will not only prevent peptic ulceration, but it will cure it in the vast majority of those afflicted. This nutrition regimen is detailed in Chapter II. It calls for *no* sugar, alcohol, caffeine (coffee, tea, chocolate or caffeine-containing soft drinks) or tobacco in any form (especially cigarettes). Also helpful and occasionally essential is the reduction to, or the maintenance of, a normal weight. Excessive fat (obesity) and overeating (gorging at meal time) can aggravate symptoms and make cure more difficult.

It isn't easy to follow this nutrition regimen, but neither is it easy to live with the pain and discomfort of "peptic ulcer" and its life-endangering complications.

Peptic ulcer is a condition which has been the subject of several most interesting epidemiological studies. There are certainly few of us in the "Western" world who have not experienced some of the symptoms of peptic ulcer, and among these are included indigestion, pain, burning, bloating, gas and heartburn. The treatment of peptic ulcer has spawned a multimillion dollar antacid industry and we are constantly bombarded via television and radio by advertisements telling us how to get relief from the nagging symptoms of this common ailment. One would think that were an easy answer available, it would long since have become general knowledge, but such is not the case. *There is an easy answer* and the following epidemiological observations should make it clear to you, even before I outline the simple method that will allow you to *cure yourself*. Keep in mind the fact that this illness kills over ten thousand persons annually in the United States alone from hemorrhage and perforation, in addition to causing untold suffering in many millions of us and you discover an extremely cogent reason for exposing the cause of this distressing and sometimes fatal affliction.

What is the cause of peptic ulcer? Is it stress? Is it the Type A personality? Is it heredity? *Absolutely not!* These may be minor influences which may increase the risk of developing peptic ulceration, but they are not the main cause. Let us examine some of the results of epidemiological research showing which populations are at risk and which are not and then consider the cause in the light of these facts.

In many parts of Africa it has been well documented that peptic ulcer is a rarity in people living on mainly coarse, unrefined carbohydrates, almost regardless of what else they may consume. However, when these populations become urbanized and begin ingesting large amounts of refined carbohydrates (especially sugar) they begin to develop peptic ulcers just as those of us on the high-sugar "Western" diet. In India we find the same situation. Those populations subsisting mainly on a diet of coarse, unrefined carbohydrates rarely develop peptic ulcers, but those ingesting large quantities of refined carbohydrates (especially sugar) develop peptic ulcers and die of the complications just as we do in the "Western" world.

What happened to the people of Europe during the stressful bombing raids of World War II? Did they develop peptic ulceration? The answer is *no*. The rationing of sugar forced them to ingest a coarse, unrefined carbohydrate diet and this protected them from developing peptic ulcers despite stress, Type A personality and despite heredity. What protected the foreign prisoners of war in Japan in World War II from developing peptic ulcers? It was the coarse, unrefined carbohydrate diet. What protected the German soldiers from developing ulcers late in the war on the Eastern Front when hundreds of thousands were losing their lives? It was the crude, coarse, unrefined carbohydrate diet which often consisted of raw vegetables dug from the ground by the soldiers themselves.

What then is the cause of peptic ulceration? Must it not be mainly due to the eating of refined foods to the almost exclusion of coarse, unrefined foods? And if this be so, why is it so? The explanation is simple.

The stomach secretes acid in the process of digestion and this is the substance that can cause inflammation and ulceration of the stomach and the beginning of the small intestine, the duodenal bulb. However, when the stomach is empty there is little or no acid present and the walls of the stomach present a thick, protective mucous lining to any acid which might be secreted, so no inflammation or ulceration can occur. Therefore, when the stomach is empty, we are safe, and healing can begin to take place if any inflammation or ulcer is present.

However, when food enters the stomach, the walls are stretched out so that the protective mucous lining is made thinner and therefore less resistant to the acid which is secreted by the stomach in response to food. If protein and fiber have been stripped from the food in the refining process, as in refined carbohydrates (especially sugar, white rice and white flour) there is then little to buffer the stomach acid and the acid begins attacking the thin, stretched stomach lining and the lining of the proximal portion of the duodenum. What would be the most dangerous food? Certainly it must be refined sugar, which calls forth the acid, contains no buffering protein to counteract the acid, and because of its lack of fiber passes quickly into the duodenum. With repeated unbuffered acid insults from refined sugar we begin to develop inflammation of the stomach and duodenal bulb and ulceration may occur. You must certainly by now know the answer to the question of how to prevent and treat peptic ulcer. Don't you agree that it is simple?

1. If you must drink sugared coffee, sugared soft drinks or eat sugary baked goods on an empty stomach, resign yourself to the eventual development of abdominal discomfort and perhaps even peptic ulceration.
2. If you must eat sugar, eat some protein with it to protect your stomach and duodenum, even a raw vegetable or fruit should suffice.

3. If your stomach is empty, it is safe and can begin healing itself.
4. If you eat under great emotional stress or overeat when you are not hungry, your stomach will tend to empty slowly and give any unbuffered acid a better and longer opportunity to cause trouble.

Prevention of Peptic Ulcer
1. The *Correct Nutrition* regimen detailed in Chapter II, which allows *no* refined carbohydrates (especially sugar, white rice and white flour) and stresses the consumption of fresh, raw or steamed vegetables and fresh, raw fruit, will prevent peptic ulceration.

Treatment and Cure of Peptic Ulcer
1. The *Correct Nutrition* regimen noted above under *Prevention of Peptic Ulcer*.
2. No alcoholic or sugared beverages.
3. No cigarettes.
4. Do not eat unless you are hungry and then only foods from the food lists in Chapter II.
5. Drink only water or skim milk if you must have something between meals.
6. Remember that your stomach and duodenal lining is healing and best protected when your stomach is empty.

Hiatal Hernia

The term, hernia, means the protrusion of an organ or tissue through a hiatus or opening. When a portion of the stomach and lower end of the esophagus pushes up into the chest cavity through the normal or slightly enlarged esophageal hiatus in the diaphragm, we have a "hiatal hernia".

These "hiatal hernias" are very common, especially in older, overweight or obese people who may have suffered from "indigestion" for years, and who have enjoyed the "better" things of life (high-sugar, high-fat diets and gourmet foods).

"Hiatal hernias" tend to be annoying rather than dangerous. The major signs and symptoms are caused by reflux of acid contents of the stomach into the esophagus causing heartburn and upper abdominal discomfort. This disagreeable reflux of bitter, acid stomach contents may reach the throat or mouth and cause burning, choking and gasping for air as it irritates the laryngeal mucosal lining and interferes with breathing.

Frequently the patients are overweight or obese, and typically the difficulty comes on during the night after overeating or after ingesting food or drink that causes them to feel that they have "indigestion" such as "gas", "bloating", or "a feeling of fullness and abdominal discomfort". They usually go to sleep, but then suddenly waken with a reflux of bitter, acid stomach contents in their throats. Many have thought they were dying of a heart attack as they choked, gagged, coughed and gasped for air.

The cause of this diaphragmatic hernia, "hiatal hernia", is the dietary indiscretions of many years, and treatment should be directed at prevention of symptoms since this condition is generally a problem, only in that it causes this disagreeable reflux of acid stomach contents.

Prevention of the reflux is simple. The nutrition regimen detailed in Chapter II combined with loss of excess weight will often bring immediate relief. In fact, avoidance of food and drink for five hours before bedtime may also prevent it completely.

Prevention of Hiatal Hernia

1. The *Correct Nutrition* regimen as detailed in Chapter II will prevent *Hiatal Hernia*, as populations subsisting mainly on coarse, natural, unrefined diets provide indisputable testimony to the fact.

Treatment of Hiatal Hernia

1. The *Correct Nutrition* regimen as detailed in Chapter II.
2. Get rid of excess weight or obesity.
3. Never gorge at mealtime.
4. Prevent acid, nocturnal reflux and heartburn by simply not eating or drinking for five hours prior to going to bed at night.

CHAPTER XI

Constipation and the Irritable Colon Syndrome

A dictionary defines "constipation" as "a condition of the bowels, marked by defective or difficult evacuation of feces". This seems technically correct, but a more enlightened definition would be "a condition of the bowels, marked by defective or difficult evacuation and caused by a diet containing too little fiber". A diet high in fiber content makes constipation virtually impossible. A high-fiber diet, such as detailed in Chapter II, will abolish constipation absolutely and completely. It will increase the bulk and weight of the stool. It will soften and normalize the stool. It will also decrease the intraluminal pressures, thus causing less chance of developing diverticulosis (outpouching pockets in the bowel wall which can become inflamed and infected). In addition, it will decrease the transit time through the colon of potentially hazardous, poisonous and other chemical products of digestion and will dilute them by means of the increased bulk of the stool.

Small, hard stools that remain long in contact with the bowel wall because of long transit time are hazardous to your health. In constipated persons, the long contact with some of the poisonous and concentrated products of digestion are implicated in the causation of cancer of the colon and irritable bowel syndrome. The grunting, straining, and pushing required to pass hard masses of feces may lead directly to the development of "hemorrhoids", and has even been listed as an indirect cause of "varicose veins" and "hiatal hernias". You should be advised that many persons encounter "sudden death" on the toilet seat, where their herculean efforts to pass a constipated stool precipitated their fatal heart attack.

"Irritable bowel syndrome" is one of the most common forms of anxiety seen in the physician's office. It is often associated with a long history of constipation, complicated by the overuse of laxatives and enemas. The history often details the relief from the abdominal pain and discomfort by the passage of small, hard constipated stools or by the manual removal of a large, hard fecal impaction.

"Constipation" and "irritable bowel syndrome" are caused by low-fiber, high-sugar diets and prevented and cured by high-fiber, low-sugar diets. The nutrition regimen detailed in Chapter II, coupled with a regular, sensible exercise program, will cure these conditions absolutely, and in a surprisingly short period of time.

Does it not seem better to cure "constipation" than to be constantly resorting to laxatives and enemas to relieve your abdominal and rectal discomfort? It is true that on a high-fiber diet, one may occasionally be made uncomfortable by a desire to pass rectal gas, but this usually becomes less and less a problem as the intestinal tract adjusts to the new program.

Ulcerative Colitis and Crohn's Disease

These often rather ill-defined diseases of the bowel are often characterized by abdominal pain and diarrhea that is frequently bloody. The specific cause is unknown and many patients must be treated by surgical excision of diseased portions of the bowel.

These afflictions may also be examples of self-induced disease and are probably preventable. The incidence of these conditions varies greatly among different populations and evidence is pointing toward improper diet as a causative agent. As a preventative and treatment measure, one should consider the correct nutrition program detailed in Chapter II.

Summary

We know from epidemiological studies that populations, which subsist mainly on coarse, natural, unrefined carbohydrate foods, do not suffer from constipation or irritable bowel syndrome, and ulcerative colitis and Crohn's disease are practically never seen. However, when these people migrate to the cities or to "Western" countries and embrace the low-fiber, high-sugar "Western" type of diet, they are likely to suffer constipation and irritable bowel syndrome, and even ulcerative colitis and Crohn's disease may afflict them.

Prevention of Constipation and Irritable Bowel Syndrome

1. The *Correct Nutrition* regimen as detailed in Chapter II, which allows *no* refined carbohydrates (especially sugar, white rice and white flour) and which stresses the consumption of large quantities of coarse, natural, fresh, raw or steamed vegetables and fresh, raw fruit, makes constipation virtually impossible and will also prevent irritable bowel syndrome.

Treatment and Cure of Constipation and Irritable Bowel Syndrome

1. Same as noted above under *Prevention of Constipation and Irritable Bowel Syndrome*.

Prevention of Ulcerative Colitis and Crohn's Disease

1. The *Correct Nutrition* regimen as detailed in Chapter II, which allows *no* refined carbohydrates (especially sugar, white rice and white flour) and which stresses the consumption of large quantities of coarse, natural, fresh, raw or steamed vegetables and fresh, raw fruit, will in all probability prevent ulcerative colitis or Crohn's disease from ever occurring.

Treatment of Ulcerative Colitis and Crohn's Disease

1. Same as noted under *Prevention of Ulcerative Coltis and Crohn's Disease*.
2. Surgery may become necessary in advanced cases.

CHAPTER XII

Hemorrhoids

"Hemorrhoids" are commonly called "piles" by the layman. They are enlargements of the blood vessels (veins) in the anal canal, the terminal portion of the bowel which lies between the rectum and the anal opening. If they are high in the anal canal (above the pectinate line) they are called internal hemorrhoids. If they lie below the pectinate line of the anal canal, they are called external hemorrhoids. Internal hemorrhoids are usually too high in the anal canal to be felt or seen by casual inspection or without a physician's instrument. They are ordinarily painless, and bleeding is the common sign of their presence. The blood is bright red in color, is found in the toilet bowl or on the toilet tissue, and often coats the outside of the stool, but is not mixed through the inner portions of the fecal mass. External hemorrhoids tend to be easily felt, plainly visible, and are generally painful, especially during the passage of a bowel movement. When hemorrhoids are thrombosed (that means when the blood in them has clotted), they become firm, sore, painful, tender, swollen masses which make defecation or straining at stool both painful and bloody.

Hemorrhoids may be caused by the constipation often accompanying tumors, pregnancy, liver disease, and other conditions which can increase the pressure in the veins that drain the anal region. However, the major contributing factor in the production of hemorrhoids is "constipation" caused by a low-fiber diet. If one does not become constipated, obviously one will not need to strain at stool and will, in all probability, never develop hemorrhoids, even should pregnancies supervene or other precipitating factors make their appearance.

The prevention of hemorrhoids is accomplished most simply by adhering to a nutrition program involving avoidance of sugar and ingestion of foods high in fiber and low in fat as detailed in Chapter II. Hemorrhoids are rare in the undeveloped regions of the world where unrefined-carbohydrate, high-fiber diets are the rule.

Pruritus Ani

The term "pruritus ani" simply means an "itching sensation around the anal opening". This "itching" may become so intense that it robs people of sleep and may cause acute embarrassment when they are caught surreptitiously scratching their "bottoms" in public. It can also cause a laundry problem. The incessant scratching can cause the undergarments to be stained to such a degree that special scrubbing of this area becomes necessary before the article is put in the washing machine. The "itching" sometimes drives people to distraction and interferes with their work as well as their sleep.

Many patients have undergone hemorrhoid surgery in a futile attempt to correct this problem. Others have used ointments, caustics, proprietary medicines and prescription drugs without lasting relief.

However, the problem is really a very simple one. A nutrition program calling for only natural unrefined carbohydrates and very little fat as detailed in Chapter II, combined with daily cleansing of the region with a mild soap and water usually abolishes the "itching" in less than a week.

One is certainly well-advised to use this method to attack any minor "itching" problem in the anal area, before seeking professional help on the premise that it might possibly be one of the odd cases with a more sinister origin.

Varicose Veins

Arteries are blood vessels which carry oxygenated blood from the heart to the tissues of the body. Veins are the thinner-walled blood vessels which return the deoxygenated blood from the body tissues to the heart.

Varicose veins are dilated enlarged veins and they are commonly seen in the lower extremities, especially in the legs and thighs.

The causes of varicose veins have in the past been thought to be due to an inherited weakness or an occupation requiring standing (clerks in stores, dentists), or in some instances tumors or pregnancy, etc. However, the anatomically reasonable explanation put forward by T.L. Cleave is quite probably the primary one. Chronic constipation with colonic stasis and loading could cause varicose veins by slight unnatural pressures on the veins draining the lower extremities whenever that individual was lying in the supine position.

However, the constipation which causes the colonic stasis and loading is easily preventable. All that is needed is the adoption of the correct nutrition regimen detailed in Chapter II. If adherence to correct nutrition is faithfully followed, there will be no constipation, no colonic stasis and loading and no unsightly or incapacitating varicose veins despite pregnancy, occupation, etc.

Varicose veins are preventable and surgery is usually only a palliative procedure.

Varicocele

The term varicocele usually refers to dilated enlarged blood vessels in the male scrotal sac. These are veins that drain the testicle. Varicocele is more common on the left side as are varicose veins in the left thigh and leg. This is due to the fact that the left portion of the colon or large bowel is more directly positioned to allow it to exert pressure on the venous drainage system of the left side of the body when there is constipation with colonic stasis and loading.

Varicocele can be prevented by avoiding constipation with its complications of colonic stasis and loading. The correct nutrition regimen detailed in Chapter II will prevent varicocele from occurring.

Pulmonary Embolism

Pulmonary embolism (pulmonary thromboembolism) is a condition which is responsible for the "sudden death" of thousands of medical, surgical and obstetrical patients every year, and in many cases it may have been *a preventable catastrophe*.

Simply put, the blood clot or thrombus often forms in the deep veins of the lower extremity or pelvis while the patient is convalescing in the supine position after surgery, on a medical service, or following an obstetrical delivery. If this blood clot breaks away and passes upward through the ever larger venous blood channels to and through the heart to the lung, it may cause "sudden death".

How may we insure against this happening to us if we are bedfast, pregnant or require surgery? Your physician will take all or most of the possible precautions against this catastrophe, but there is one thing that you can do that might be crucial. By adhering to a correct nutrition regimen you will be making certain that you have no constipation with colonic stasis and loading. If your colon or large bowel is relatively empty while you are bedfast, during surgery or delivery, and during convalesence there will be less tendency to slow venous blood flow from the extremities and therefore less chance of developing a blood clot and of having a fatal pulmonary embolus.

Summary

Hemorrhoids, varicose veins and varicocele are caused by increased venous pressures, and pulmonary embolism is due to thrombi formed in the presence of venous stasis, but all are due indirectly to constipation with its resulting colonic stasis and loading.

Constipation is almost invariably caused by a low-fiber diet which results in an increased transit time for body wastes passing through the intestinal tract. This increased transit time results in loading of the colon with abnormally large and heavy amounts of fecal material which tend to be much more dry and hard than normal. The *lack of fiber*, which is responsible for the accumulation of these slow-moving, relatively dry, fecal masses, is held to be the cause of sluggish movement or colonic stasis. It is also the cause of the absorption of large amounts of water from the slow-moving fecal masses and consequently the colonic loading or accumulation. This colonic stasis and loading is most pronounced in the rectum, sigmoid and cecal portions of the colon, and not surprisingly these are the regions where most cancers of the colon occur.

The stasis and loading of the cecum and distal colon are especially capable of exerting pressure on the veins draining the lower parts of the body whenever the individual is in the supine position. This is especially true on the left side where the colon lies directly against the veins draining the left lower extremity and testicle. Pressure can also be exerted on the veins draining the right lower extremity by a loaded cecum when the person is in a supine position, but because of anatomical conditions it is somewhat less likely. Therefore we find varicocele and varicose veins of the extremities more frequently on the left than on the right. Heavy fecal masses in the colon, by pressing on the veins draining the lower extremities when we are supine, can increase the pressure in the veins, damaging the valves and creating the large, unsightly, dilated veins that we refer to as varicose veins. Varicocele is formed in the identical manner by pressure on the veins draining the testicle.

Hemorrhoids are caused by the loading of the rectum, which not only interferes with the venous drainage of the anal canal over long periods of time but subjects these veins to intense pressures during the straining at stool that becomes necessary to evacuate large, hard fecal masses.

Pulmonary embolism is also the result of colonic loading due to constipation, though more indirectly. The pressure on the veins draining the lower extremities when the patient is supine tends to cause venous stasis which may give rise to thrombus formation in the leg veins. This is a major reason why patients who are bedfast on medical wards or post-operative on surgical or obstetrical wards must not be allowed to have their venous drainage from the lower extremities slowed by pressures of colonic loading, for thrombi may form in the veins that are capable of producing fatal pulmonary embolism.

Prevention of Hemorrhoids (Piles)

1. The *Correct Nutrition* regimen as detailed in Chapter II, which allows *no* refined carbohydrates (especially sugar, white rice and white flour) and stresses the consumption of large quantities of fresh, raw or steamed vegetables and fresh, raw fruit, will prevent the development of hemorrhoids even during pregnancy.

Treatment and Cure of Hemorrhoids

1. Same as listed above under *Prevention*.
2. Surgery if indicated, but prevent recurrence by the *Correct Nutrition* regimen detailed in Chapter II.

Prevention of Pruritus Ani

1. The *Correct Nutrition* regimen as detailed in Chapter II, which allows *no* refined carbohydrates (especially sugar, white rice and white flour) and which stresses the consumption of large quantities of fresh, raw or steamed vegetables and fresh, raw fruit, makes constipation virtually impossible and will also prevent Pruritus Ani.

Treatment and Cure of Pruritus Ani

1. Same as listed above under *Prevention*.
2. Wash anal area with warm soapy water after each bowel movement until "itching" has completely disappeared.

Prevention of Varicose Veins

1. The *Correct Nutrition* regimen as detailed in Chapter II, which allows *no* refined carbohydrates (especially sugar, white rice and white flour) and stresses the consumption of large quantities of fresh, raw or steamed vegetables and fresh, raw fruit, can prevent the formation of varicose veins even in pregnancy by preventing constipation with its accompanying colonic stasis and loading.

Prevention of Varicocele

1. The *Correct Nutrition* regimen as detailed in Chapter II, which allows *no* refined carbohydrates (especially sugar, white rice and white flour) and stresses the consumption of large quantities of fresh, raw or steamed vegetables and fresh, raw fruit, will prevent the formation of varicocele by decreasing the pressure of the colon on the left gonadal vein when the patient is in the supine position.

Treatment and Cure of Varicocele

1. Same as listed above under *Prevention of Varicocele*.
2. Surgery if indicated.

Prevention of Pulmonary Embolism

1. Prevention of pulmonary embolism can be accomplished by preventing constipation with its colonic stasis and loading in all surgical and obstetrical patients and all bedridden patients whether on medical wards or in convalescent areas. The pressure of a loaded colon on the veins draining the lower extremities while patients are in the supine position for long periods of time must be avoided.
2. Prevention therefore depends on the *Correct Nutrition* regimen as detailed in Chapter II. It allows *no* refined carbohydrates (especially sugar, white rice and white flour) and stresses the consumption of large quantities of fresh, raw or steamed vegetables and fresh, raw fruit.
3. Enemas or laxatives will be absolutely necessary if the bedfast, supine patient *will not* or *can not* take the *Correct Nutrition* regimen.

CHAPTER XIII

Diverticulitis

Diverticulitis simply means inflammation of a diverticulum or of more than one diverticulum. These outpouchings or sacs protrude outward from the bowel wall, each like a tiny, thin-walled appendix. They are apparently caused by the increased intraluminal pressures which accompany constipation and straining at stool. These tiny ballooned-out sacs in the bowel are most frequently found in the sigmoid colon, which is the portion of the colon just above the rectum.

These very small diverticula or sacs occur in probably 10% of people over 50 in the United States, and the incidence then increases with age. Diverticulosis is the disease condition characterized by the presence of these ballooned-out sacs protruding from the bowel wall, and inflammation of one or more of these sacs constitutes diverticulitis.

Diverticulitis is caused by the "Western" diet that is low in fiber and high in sugar. This diet not only causes the diverticula to form in the first place, but provides the perfect milieu or medium for the infection of these thin-walled outpouchings or sacs. The bacterial flora of the bowel is changed by the high-sugar diet to promote not only diverticulitis, but appendicitis as well. Bacteria from the colon invade the tissues of these thin-walled sacs causing infection, inflammation and even abscess formation and peritonitis. Diverticulitis may frequently simulate a left-sided appendicitis. The most usual symptoms are lower abdominal pain, made worse by defecation.

Bleeding or even massive hemorrhage into the colon is another complication of diverticulitis. The blood vessels supplying the thin-walled, ballooned-out sacs are poorly protected and more subject to damage by hard, constipated stool.

Again, the prevention of diverticulosis is accomplished by adhering to the high-fiber diet detailed in Chapter II. Any condition caused by constipation can be prevented by the high-fiber diet that is free of refined carbohydrates and low in fat, as illustrated by statistics showing diverticulitis to be rare to unknown in the primitive and developing countries where a high-fiber diet is the rule, and a very common disease in the United States and other developed countries where the low-fiber diet takes precedence.

Appendicitis

Appendicitis means inflammation of the appendix and, as we all know, appendicitis is a life-threatening illness and is a surgical emergency. The disease is extremely common in "Western" populations and urban communities throughout the world, but it is extremely uncommon in remote rural areas and in primitive societies. The tremendous differences in incidence seem to parallel the consumption of refined versus unrefined carbohydrates. Where the population consumes a low-fiber diet of refined carbohydrates (sugar, white rice and white flour), the incidence of appendicitis will be high.

Therefore, if you wish to prevent the occurrence of appendicitis in you or your family, you have only to adopt the correct nutrition regimen detailed in Chapter II. *Appendicitis is a preventable disease.*

Summary

Diverticulosis, diverticulitis and appendicitis are three more illnesses which are seldom seen in populations which subsist mainly on coarse, unrefined carbohydrate diets that are high in fiber and low in refined sugar. However, when these people migrate to cities or to countries where there is high consumption of refined sugar and the fiber content of the diet is low, they become at risk of developing these afflictions if they embrace the low-fiber, high-sugar diet of the new environment.

As stated previously, diverticulosis occurs in probably 10% of people over 50 in the United States, and the incidence increases with age, or one might say the incidence increases as the length of time on a low-fiber diet increases. The method of prevention of diverticulosis should by now be quite obvious to you, *Correct Nutrition*.

Inflammation of a diverticulum or of several diverticula is called diverticulitis and inflammation of the appendix is called appendicitis. These diseases were rare until refined carbohydrates and improved economic conditions spawned the low-fiber, high-sugar diet typical of that of the "Western" world. When colonic stasis and loading occur as a result of the constipation produced by the low-fiber diet, and when the normal bacterial flora begin to multiply so much more rapidly and wildly in an intestinal tract loaded with an undigested excess of refined sugar, we encounter a situation where the normal body defense mechanisms may become overwhelmed, and serious infections in the most vulnerable areas in the regions of greatest colonic stasis are apt to occur. These most vulnerable areas of greatest colonic stasis are any small diverticula in the left lower colon and the appendix in the cecal region. Thus diverticulitis and appendicitis have become common diseases in the "Western" world and will become common in any population which embraces the low-fiber, high-sugar, "Western" type of diet.

Prevention of Diverticulosis and Diverticulitis
1. The *Correct Nutrition* regimen as detailed in Chapter II, which allows *no* refined carbohydrates (especially sugar, white rice and white flour) and stresses the consumption of large quantities of fresh, raw or steamed vegetables and fresh, raw fruit, will prevent both diverticulosis and diverticulitis.

Treatment of Diverticulosis and Diverticulitis
1. Same as listed above under *Prevention*.
2. Surgery if indicated.

Prevention of Appendicitis

1. The *Correct Nutrition* regimen as detailed in Chapter II, which allows *no* refined carbohydrates (especially sugar, white rice and white flour) and stresses the consumption of large quantities of fresh, raw or steamed vegetables and fresh, raw fruit, can prevent appendicitis from occurring in any but extremely rare instances.

Treatment and Cure of Appendicitis

1. Surgical.

CHAPTER XIV

Cancer

It has been seriously suggested that "as many as 90% of all cancers may be preventable, once the causative environmental factors are isolated and their relationships to the various forms of cancer are completely understood". In the light of the following discussion, you may indeed decide that the above suggestion, radical as it may seem at first glance, may in fact be very close to the mark.

Many cancers show marked differences in prevalance throughout the world, and that seems to indicate that they may be preventable. When people migrate from areas of low incidence to regions where the rate of occurrence of a certain form of cancer is high, we might expect that after they had become acclimated to the new environment, that they and their offspring would become more susceptible to the development of this cancer, if indeed environmental factors exert major effects. This is exactly what occurs in many instances.

Cancer of the breast, our leading cause of death from cancer in U.S. women, shows dramatic differences in world-wide distribution which seem to be modified by immigration. Japan has a death rate from this cancer that is much lower than that of the United States, but the incidence rises in Japanese women and their children who migrate to the United States. Diet has been implicated as a possible cause of breast cancer, and one study showed that among the higher socioeconomic classes in Japan, this form of malignancy occurred 8 times more frequently than among the lower classes. Another study has found that Seventh-Day Adventist vegetarians have lower rates of breast cancer than does the general population. Still other research indicates a higher rate of this disease in the overweight and obese than in their peers.

Cancer of the prostate gland is 6 times more common in the United States than in Japan, but the reverse is true of gastric malignancy. Gastric (stomach) cancer has an incidence in Japan that is 8 times that found in this country. These statistics illustrate quite well some of the dramatic differences in the incidence of various cancers throughout the world among different populations.

When the above findings are considered, along with the fact that over 20% of all deaths in the United States are due to malignant tumors, and with the statistic that shows cancer to be a leading cause of death in this country, second only to heart disease, one can easily understand why there has been a tremendous surge of interest in investigations of dietary and other environmental influences on the many and diverse forms of these malignant afflictions.

Cancer of the colon appears to be absolutely preventable if one adheres to a high-fiber nutrition regimen such as is detailed in Chapter II. However, accompanying the high amount of fiber in the diet is the restriction of refined carbohydrates, fats and processed and packaged foods with their chemical additives and preservatives, and these restrictions may offer protection from malignancy in addition to that brought about by the fiber.

Cancer of the lung, the leading cause of cancer deaths in men and the third leading cause in women, is another form of cancer related to environmental factors. Cigarette smoking has been implicated as a major causative factor in the production of this malignant disease for more than three decades.

With the present state of our knowledge of environmental influences which affect the incidence of cancer, we would be well advised to follow the nutrition regimen detailed in this book. Cigarettes, caffeine, and many chemical food additives and preservatives would be eliminated, and we would enjoy the protection against a host of illnesses, including degenerative coronary artery disease and many forms of cancer, afforded by this high-fiber, low-fat diet, composed mainly of carbohydrate foods in their natural state.

Prevention of Cancer

We do not know how to prevent all "Cancer", but we do know that environmental factors are involved in many instances, probably as many as 90%.

If we all stopped smoking cigarettes, the incidence of *Cancer of the Lung* would decrease markedly, and *Cancer of the Lung* is the leading cause of cancer deaths in men and the third leading cause of cancer deaths in women.

If we all became vegetarians, it seems that *Cancer of the Breast* would show a marked drop and this is the leading cause of cancer death in U.S. women.

If we all went over to a high-fiber diet, we would see very little *Cancer of the Colon* or *Cancer of the Rectum*, and these at present account for the second leading cause of cancer deaths in both women and men in the United States.

If we all followed the *Correct Nutrition* regimen as detailed in Chapter II, we might easily eliminate the majority of cancers now responsible for the three leading causes of death from cancer in both women and men in the United States today.

CHAPTER XV

Cancer of the Colon

Cancer is second only to heart disease as the leading cause of death in the United States for both men and women, and it accounts for over 20% of deaths from all causes.

Cancer of the colon and rectum is one of the most common of all malignant tumors, and it is second only to cancer of the lung as the leading cause of death from cancer in men and is second only to cancer of the breast in women.

The signs and symptoms of "cancer of the colon" (including the rectum, which is the lower portion of the colon), include change in bowel habit (especially change in caliber of the stool and an uncomfortable sensation that bowel evacuation is not complete), bleeding (either occult or grossly visible and mixed throughout the fecal material, as opposed to merely coating the outside of the fecal mass), pain, anemia (with pallor and ease of fatigue), and weight loss and anorexia (loss of appetite).

Digital examination and x-ray are excellent diagnostic procedures and visual inspection of the inner walls of the colon with long, pliable optical instruments can bring the vast majority of these neoplasms into direct view. Once discovered, surgical excision and chemotherapy can cure the colon and rectal cancers of many patients, but *"Cancer of the Colon"* is a *"Preventable Disease"*.

Epidemiological studies show that cancer of the colon varies as much as 10-fold in incidence among different populations, and that when people migrate from regions with low incidence to regions of high incidence, they are at increased risk as they become acclimated to the radical changes from their high-fiber, natural-food diet to the low-fiber, high-sugar, processed-food diet of the new culture.

Prevention of "cancer of the colon" is almost guaranteed by the nutrition regimen detailed in Chapter II, combined with the regular exercise program designed to further aid bowel evacuation and further prevent the degenerative atherosclerosis of blood vessels supplying the colon. In the absence of atherosclerosis, the arteries supply the colon with adequate amounts of oxygenated arterial blood, and this in itself is a further deterrent to the formation of colon malignancies.

Prevention of Cancer of the Colon and Cancer of the Rectum

1. The *Correct Nutrition* regimen as detailed in Chapter II, which allows *no* refined carbohydrates (especially sugar, white rice and white flour) and stresses the consumption of large quantities of fresh, raw or steamed vegetables and fresh, raw fruit, can prevent cancer of the colon and cancer of the rectum as epidemiological research has proven.

CHAPTER XVI

Gallstones (Cholelithiasis)

The word "cholelithiasis" simply means gallstones. It is estimated that 10% of all adults in the United States have gallstones, and that by age 70, the prevalence has risen to 30%. We are not absolutely certain about the causes of these stones, but their relationship to our refined-carbohydrate, low-fiber, high-fat diet seems undeniable. There are many thousands of surgical operations performed each year for the removal of gallstones and the problems they create. Many of the crises they precipitate are life-threatening ones. The morbidity associated with gallstones is staggering, and we are talking about *a preventable disease*.

It has been estimated that 50% of gallstones remain "silent". They apparently may cause few or no symptoms throughout the patient's lifetime and may be discovered only incidentally at an operation for some other condition or at autopsy. When gallstones do cause problems, the symptoms may be quite mild, such as vague abdominal pains, intolerance of fat or greasy food, nausea or vomiting. However, gallstones can create serious difficulties and life-threatening emergencies. Severe pain, tenderness in the right upper abdomen, chills, fever and jaundice are some of the more common indications of gallstone-provoked gallbladder disease of a more serious nature, and the long-term irritative effects of gallstones have been indicted as a causative agent in cancer of the gallbladder, a relatively uncommon disease.

Why does one develop gallstones? As we stated previously, we are not absolutely certain, but the major contributing cause is, in all probability, the "Western" diet with its high-sugar, low-fiber and high-fat content with its accompanying excessive weight and obesity.

The simplest solution to the problem of forming gallstones would appear to be the institution of a high-fiber, low-fat diet with no refined carbohydrates and the elimination of any excessive fat or obesity. There is even some evidence that gallstones may somehow dissolve or disappear, given long periods of time on high-fiber, low-fat diets with no refined sugar. The nutrition regimen detailed in Chapter II, combined with a judiciously-chosen regular exercise program will provide more than adequate insurance against the formation of gallstones and many other degenerative conditions as well.

Cholecystitis

Cholecystitis means inflammation of the gallbladder with or without gallstones. If we look at the incidence of this disease in developed countries, we find it to be high. However, among people living under relatively primitive conditions and eating unrefined foods, we find practically no gallstones or inflammatory disease of the gallbladder.

Cholecystitis (inflammation of the gallbladder), appendicitis (inflammation of the appendix), diverticulitis (inflammation of diverticula of the bowel), and pyelitis (inflammation of the kidney pelvis) seem to be common diseases in societies consuming large quanitities of refined sugars and almost unknown in cultures ingesting only unrefined carbohydrates.

The prevention of gallbladder disease would seem to be correct nutrition. The correct nutrition regimen outlined in Chapter II should prevent both gallstone formation and infection with inflammation of the gallbladder. *These conditions are mainly preventable.*

Prevention of Gallstones and Cholecystitis
   1. The *Correct Nutrition* regimen as detailed in Chapter II, which allows *no* refined carbohydrates (especially sugar, white rice and white flour) and stresses the consumption

of large quantities of fresh, raw or steamed vegetables and fresh, raw fruit, can prevent the formation of gallstones and can create a milieu in which infection and inflammation of the gallbladder (cholecystitis) will rarely ever occur.

CHAPTER XVII

Osteoporosis

Osteoporosis is a disease characterized by a demineralization, thinning and weakening of bone, so that even slight or minor injuries may cause bones to break (fracture).

The condition is very common in postmenopausal women and in both sexes after age 60. However, the incidence is always higher in females, even in the very elderly. Most of these patients appear to be otherwise well or healthy, but their decreased bone density creates problems. Vertebral fractures (often painless) may cause shortening of the spine with a decrease in the individual's vertical height. These patients often complain of vague back pain, and in postmenopausal women, a "dowager's hump" may be evidenced. Rib fracture, after relatively minor trauma, is another frequent complication.

More than 80% of the 1,000,000 fractures that occur every year in women over the age of 50 are due to osteoporosis, and most of the 200,000 hip fractures in the U.S. every year also involve this condition. The acute care alone is costing us over a billion dollars annually.

The major causes of osteoporosis are lack of exercise and lack of sufficient calcium in the diet, although hormone deficiency plays some role.

We can produce local osteoporosis simply by immobilizing a limb in a plaster cast. Generalized osteoporosis occurs when we immobilize the entire individual in a body cast or if a person is bedridden. We can also produce osteoporosis experimentally by feeding a diet deficient in calcium. This certainly indicates that exercise and high-calcium diets may be the most important preventatives. The nutrition regimen recommended in this book, combined with a judiciously-constructed exercise program can solve the problem of prevention of osteoporosis and should be the treatment of choice, with the addition of special emphasis on the ingestion of high-calcium foods.

Degenerative Joint Disease

Obesity is one of the major contributing causes of chronic degenerative disease of the weight-bearing joints, and millions of overweight patients are crowding physicians' offices, seeking relief from the pain brought on by degenerative arthritis in the back, hip and knee-joints.

The excessively-fat individual is constantly subjecting the weight-bearing joints to abnormal stresses and strains which gradually grind and hammer them into painful and comparatively useless arthritic wreckage.

The nutrition and exercise programs detailed in this book can be used to correct the obesity and prevent this kind of joint disease. *Degenerative joint disease is preventable.*

Jogging Injuries

Orthopedic problems dealing with jogging injuries include sprains, strains, stress fractures, tendonitis and damage to joints, especially the weight-bearing ones. These traumas are usually incurred by persons who are overweight or obese, or by individuals whose jogging activities are inappropriate for their age and physical fitness, or by those who may know better but push themselves, because of false pride and obstinacy, beyond the limits of their capabilities.

Summary

Osteoporosis, degenerative joint disease and most jogging injuries are preventable and so is the often associated excess of fat or obesity, if one adheres to the correct nutrition regimen and a regular, well-monitored exercise program that is tailored to the individual's unique capabilities and needs. The high-calcium, high-fiber diet of unrefined carbohydrates combined with strenuous daily exercise will prevent most osteoporosis and degenerative joint disease; and a majority of the invalids hobbling about with jogging injuries could have prevented their disabilities by getting rid of their excess fat and engaging in an appropriate exercise program that was within their capabilities and was suited to their ages and stages of physical fitness. Those overweight individuals who waddle about, ruining their hip-joints, knee-joints, and other weight-bearing joints as well, are becoming prime candidates for surgical replacement of these joints by artificial ones. In the interim, they suffer the painful agonies of arthritic, degenerative joint disease which is preventable if a correct nutrition program is entered in time to correct the osteoporosis and obesity and forestall the damage.

Prevention of Osteoporosis
1. The *Correct Nutrition* regimen as detailed in Chapter II, which allows *no* refined carbohydrates (especially sugar, white rice and white flour) and stresses the consumption of large quantities of fresh, raw or steamed vegetables and fresh, raw fruit, is the preferred diet.
2. Special emphasis should be placed on the "high-calcium" containing foods from the "Food Lists" in Chapter II.
3. Eight ounces (one glass) of skim milk, three times a day provides over 800 mg. of calcium daily.
4. A rapid (thirty-minute), two-mile walk daily, seven days a week is needed to stress the weight-bearing bones and thus prevent osteoporotic changes.
5. Some exercising of the upper extremities for at least three minutes daily with weights might well be added to the exercise program.

Treatment and Cure of Osteoporosis
1. Same as detailed above for *Prevention of Osteoporosis*.

Prevention of Degenerative Joint Disease and Jogging Injuries

1. Prevention or cure of obesity and the loss of all excess weight will minimize any tendency toward joint injury during exercise.

2. The *Correct Nutrition* regimen detailed in Chapter II, combined with a thorough understanding of Chapters III and IV on exercise and obesity, will enable one to lose any excess weight and to maintain a normal weight.

3. Sports and exercise programs, that are appropriate for the individuals' capabilities and suited to their ages and stages of physical fitness, are the only ones that should be allowed or chosen.

4. Stretching exercises should precede engagement in any sport or exercise program.

CHAPTER XVIII

Arthritis

"Arthritis" means inflammation of joints. The term is usually used to refer to diseases characterized by inflammatory changes involving the joint capsule and the internal structures which include bone, cartilage and the synovium or inner lining. These changes are usually accompanied by deformity. However, when no evident inflammatory process is present, the diseased and deformed joint may be more properly termed an "arthropathy".

The terms "arthritis" and "arthropathy" encompass so many different illnesses that space does not allow even a short discussion of each. In fact, few of us would be interested and most would be bored and lost in detail if forced to read as much as a simple listing of these maladies.

However, we can all easily understand that obesity can cause "arthritis" in the weight-bearing joints by the constant stress, grinding and pounding to which the joints are subjected, day after day and year after year. Much of this can of course be prevented by getting rid of the excess fat with a correct nutrition program.

There are other forms of degenerative "arthritis", including "rheumatoid arthritis" and some of its variants, that respond favorably to both an improved nutrition regimen and a judicious or prudent exercise or physical therapy program that is uniquely designed to fit that individual's situation.

"Rheumatoid arthritis" is a chronic degenerative disease which causes characteristic crippling deformities, and its cause is unknown. We do appreciate, however, that the institution of a correct nutrition regimen of mainly unrefined carbohydrates which will be low in fat and high in fiber should be the first step in both prevention and treatment. This correct nutrition approach will help in one respect by eliminating any tendency toward constipation. It will increase the rate of passage of food through the intestinal tract and thus allow less time for absorption of noxious chemical materials. It will also provide less time for potentially-harmful products of digestion to remain in contact with the intestinal lining. In addition, we should be made aware that the exercise or physical therapy program will improve the arterial blood supply to the damaged joints, and that the low-fat diet will aid the circulation by preventing sludging and slowing of blood flow through the tiny blood vessels nourishing the diseased tissues.

Correct nutrition and judicious exercise of joints have more to offer the arthritic than any other treatment mode.

Nonarticular Rheumatism

"Rheumatism" is a common term for the affliction distinguished by pain, tenderness and stiffness in muscles and structures surrounding the joints. The pain is often accompanied by limitation of motion that tends to be more marked in the morning on waking or after spending relatively long periods of time in one position. The stiffness and limitation of motion usually show some improvement after stretching, passive movements or mild exercise.

It has been estimated that approximately 30% of all patients attending "arthritis clinics" have "nonarticular rheumatism". They have pain, tenderness, soreness and stiffness that makes their lives miserable. In addition to these cases of "rheumatism", there are millions upon millions of people who suffer in comparative silence and who attribute their aches, pains and stiffness to the aging process. They often resort to proprietary or patent medicines for relief, and in so doing, not infrequently cause medical problems of a more serious nature than the "rheumatism". Inflammation of the stomach (gastritis) and anemia are two of the more common sequelae.

How does one prevent or cure "rheumatism"? The safe and simple method is to adhere to a correct nutrition regimen and begin a well-designed program of regular exercise (walking is best). The good nutritional regimen will ensure that easy, rapid progress of the contents of the large bowel (colon) will take place. Soft, bulky, regular, natural bowel movements (unassisted by laxatives) will begin to occur daily or even more frequently. Harmful substances will be speedily and efficiently removed from the body and poisoning of the entire system may be eliminated. This nutrition regimen will, if followed faithfully, eliminate from our diet many of the possibly-harmful chemical additives and preservatives that may be found in processed and packaged foods, some of which must certainly be detrimental to our health.

The exercise or physical therapy program will improve the arterial blood supply to the rheumatic muscles and the connective and supporting tissues surrounding the joints. Of course, an exercise program may be unnecessary for those who perform hard, sustained physical labor about the home or at the workplace. However, to avoid the degenerative diseases or to treat them, one should engage in a relatively strenuous form of sustained physical activity for at least 30 minutes twice a day. Relatively rapid walking is the best exercise for this purpose, but many will need their physician's permission and advice prior to entering such an activity and will be compelled to build up their strength and stamina slowly and carefully before engaging in strenuous 30-minute walks.

It should require no more than six months of this nutrition and exercise treatment to bring immeasurable relief to most sufferers from "rheumatism" and to many tormented by the ravages of some forms of arthritis.

Gout

"Gout" is a form of arthritis that was described as early as the 5th century B.C., and actually occurs in various forms and is not a single disease entity. We can characterize it, however, as an acute, excruciatingly painful arthritis with a peak age of onset between the fourth and fifth decades. It has a tendency to recur at intervals with asymptomatic periods intervening between acute attacks.

The initial attack of gouty arthritis usually subsides spontaneously after a few days or weeks, but it tapers off much more quickly if medical treatment is instituted. Almost 50% of initial attacks involve the great toe, but often an ankle, heel, knee or wrist may be affected, and the inflamed joints can be swollen, painful and exquisitely tender.

There are many drugs that are useful in the treatment of "gout", but preventative medicine, in the form of a low-sugar, low-fat, high-fiber diet coupled with the avoidance of alcoholic beverages (especially beer, ale and wine), is the treatment of first choice.

We can prevent "gout" or gouty arthritis from occurring by following the nutrition regimen detailed in Chapter II, and entering a regular exercise program, specifically designed to fit the individual's unique situation.

Unfortunately, many persons refuse to change their life-style (dietary habits and sedentary practices). They prefer to submit to these exquisitely painful episodes of acute gouty arthritis. They would rather undergo the expensive, time-consuming medical examinations, x-rays and blood tests and ingest the potentially-hazardous medications.

Some undoubtedly revel in the pity and sympathy they receive from family, friends and colleagues during their hours and days of suffering. Perhaps the sympathy fully compensates them for the agony, expense and time lost from work. However, correct nutrition, coupled with a regular exercise program provides a perfect preventative. Thus, the individual with enough moral fiber and enough respect and consideration for the family can usually be freed from this acutely painful malady simply by changing the eating, drinking and sedentary habits.

The correct nutrition program detailed in Chapter II, outlines a diet of unrefined carbohydrates that is low in fat and sugar and high in fiber and a perfect preventative for gout.

What is the cure for "Gout"? Sir John Abernethy's well-known reply to the question was, "Live on sixpence a day, and *earn* it." He was describing a low-fat, high-fiber diet of unrefined carbohydrates combined with strenuous exercise.

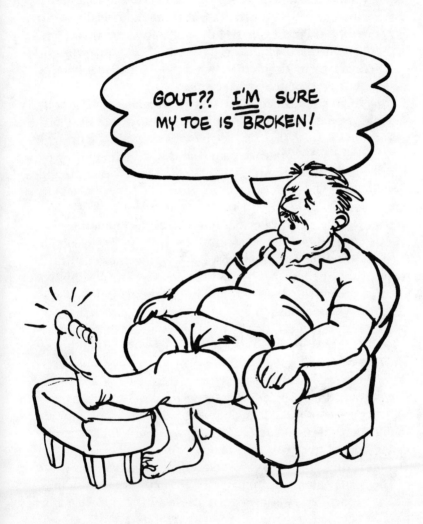

ILLUSTRATION XVIII-1

Prevention of much Arthritis, Nonarticular Rheumatism and Gout

1. The *Correct Nutrition* regimen as detailed in Chapter II, which allows *no* refined carbohydrates (especially sugar, white rice and white flour) or alcoholic beverages and which stresses the consumption of large quantities of fresh, raw or steamed vegetables and fresh, raw fruit, is the best preventative measure.

2. The *Exercise Program* as detailed in Chapter III which includes a rapid (thirty-minute), two-mile walk daily, seven days a week also contributes much to the prevention of these illnesses.

Treatment of Arthritis, Nonarticular Rheumatism and Gout

1. The *Correct Nutrition* regimen as detailed in Chapter II and noted above under *Prevention*.

2. An *Exercise Program* judiciously designed for the unique situation of the specific patient and noted above under *Prevention*.

3. Only the medication prescribed and monitored by your physician should be used.

CHAPTER XIX

Dental Caries

"Dental caries" literally means "tooth decay". This is the most widespread disease in the United States today, and in some regions the incidence is as high as 90%. Among primitive and developing country populations, excellent teeth are the rule and the deterioration of teeth in the United States can be easily correlated to the increase in the consumption of refined sugars and soft, carbohydrate foods. This gives rise to the clever remark, "teeth don't die, we kill them."

Tooth decay, with the formation of cavities, is the principal cause of loss of teeth up to 30 years of age, and is characterized by a destruction of the teeth by bacterial growth, aided and expedited by the refined sugars used in candy bars, soft drinks, ice cream and baked goods.

Dentists have been preaching against refined sugar for years as the primary reason for tooth decay. If we wish to avoid cavities and preserve our teeth for old age, we must consider good nutrition as being even more important than regular brushing. This is not to denigrate the necessity of regular cleaning of the teeth, but more to emphasize the protective contribution of good nutrition. Mr. Weston A. Price pointed out in 1950 that dental decay becomes rampant wherever a civilized refined diet overtakes an erstwhile healthy race.

The recommended food lists in the nutrition regimen outlined in Chapter II include the unrefined, natural raw vegetables and fruits that are so sorely needed, and omit all of the foods that contribute so flagrantly to the wanton destruction of teeth. May I reiterate once more? "Teeth don't die, we kill them."

Summary

Dental Caries and Periodontal Disease

Dental caries and periodontal disease are diseases of civilized societies, and epidemiological studies have shown that where populations live primitively on mainly coarse, natural, unrefined vegetables and fruit or subsist, as do Eskimoes in remote areas, mainly on meat and fat, the incidence of dental caries and periodontal disease is extremely low. However, when refined sugar is introduced to these societies, dental caries and periodontal disease become rampant. If a population has a high rate of consumption of refined carbohydrates, there will be a high incidence of dental caries and periodontal disease. The tooth decay can be directly related to the sugars which stick to the teeth and form a perfect medium to support the bacteria which destroy the teeth. All parents should understand that if they feed their babies with formulas sweetened with sucrose, give them sugar water, or quiet them with sugared pacifiers, they can destroy their infants' teeth. The parents must also be aware that if their children are allowed to eat candy bars and sugared cereals, they are being put at risk of tooth decay. Of course sugar can and does also destroy the teeth of adults. What causes periodontal disease with resulting receding gums, pyorrhea and loss of teeth? Populations who do not have access to soft, refined carbohydrates do not have this disease. This is because they must of necessity chew tough, coarse, raw, unprocessed, unrefined foods. The chewing of these unrefined foods stimulates and cleanses the teeth and stimulates the gums, keeping the gums firm and healthy and preventing periodontal problems.

Prevention of Dental Caries and Periodontal Disease

1. The *Correct Nutrition* regimen as detailed in Chapter II prevents dental caries through the restriction of sugar and white flour and the cleansing of the teeth in the process of chewing the fresh, raw fruit and the fresh, raw or steamed vegetables.
2. The chewing of tough, raw vegetables and fruits not only cleanses the teeth but stimulates the teeth and gums and

prevents periodontal disease with its sequelae of receding gums and pyorrhea.

Acne

"Acne" is a skin eruption that is one of the curses of the teenager's existence. At least 75% of both boys and girls exhibit some signs of acne at puberty. It has been described as "the classic stigma of adolescence". The inflamed lesions often become pustular and cystic and the affliction may persist beyond the second decade. Severe scarring can cause ugly disfigurement. That this inflammatory condition of the sebaceous glands of the skin is influenced by male hormones (androgenic) is illustrated by the facts that eunuchs do not develop acne, and testosterone causes the lesions to worsen.

It has long been known that infection of the lesions, by the usual bacterial flora found on the skin, responds in many cases to some of the antibiotics. It is also true that diet has often been implicated as a generating agent.

However, only recently have we been aware that the correct diet alone could not only prevent new lesions, but cause established ones to recede. The nutrition regimen detailed in Chapter II, coupled with a regular exercise program, brings immeasureable relief to these unhappy suffers often within 6 months time with remission and even complete disappearance in some.

Why do so many physicians persist in claiming that diet has nothing to do with acne? This condition is not a problem in populations living primitively on unrefined foods, but acne becomes a problem in any society that embraces the high-sugar, low-fiber, high-fat "Western" type of diet.

Prevention of Acne
1. The *Correct Nutrition* regimen detailed in Chapter II combined with a daily exercise program may prevent acne almost completely in almost any teenager.

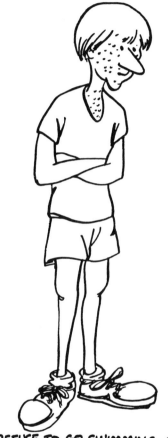

I REFUSE TO GO SWIMMING OR
PLAY BASKETBALL IF I HAVE TO
TAKE OFF MY SHIRT!

ILLUSTRATION XIX-1

Treatment and Cure of Acne

  1. Same as listed above for *Prevention of Acne*.

The Hyperactive Child

The "hyperactive child" constitutes an enigma which may never be fully explained. They are difficult to handle, high-strung, and seemingly in constant motion and in constant mischief. They create tremendous problems for themselves, their playmates, their families, their teachers and sometimes their entire communities.

Why are these children hyperactive? Why are they so different? The answers are far from clear and generally incomplete and unsatisfactory. Many of the parents are driven to absolute distraction. Is this a biochemical problem? Could certain food additives or preservatives play a poisoning type of role to which that particular child is uniquely susceptible? Could some substance such as caffeine, which is found in chocolate and many soft drinks, be a part of the problem? The scientific community has yet to provide specific answers, but we do have a method of bringing about tremendous change for the better in many of these children. Some of these children will show remarkable improvement in their behavior patterns, simply by putting them on the correct nutrition program which consists mainly of the natural, complex unrefined carbohydrates and which is low in fat. The diet should avoid refined sugar and all products which contain it. There should be as nearly as possible no canned, packaged or other processed foods containing chemical additives or preservatives. Caffeine in any form is eliminated, and meat is restricted to low-fat products, and is provided no more frequently than four times per week. Only skim milk and water are offered as beverages, but the child is encouraged to drink as much and as frequently as desired.

It is difficult to force many of these children into this eating pattern. Many will go on hunger-strikes, will obtain forbidden foods surreptitiously if any is about the house, will wheedle food from friends and neighbors, and may even take money from a mother's purse to purchase "junk" food at the nearest outlet. But if the parents have the willpower and moral fiber to hold out, if they are desperate enough, if they love the child sufficiently to realize that they are doing what is best for the child, and for themselves, in the long run they will find that they have a more normal acting child and the improved behavior will be a source of pleasure to all those who have suffered so severely in the past, especially the unfortunate little boy or girl.

The nutrition regimen to follow, to bring about this remarkable behavioral change, is detailed in Chapter II.

When the hyperactive child has been found not to have hearing defect, visual defect, etc. that might account for its abnormal behavior, we would suggest that one must search for an environmental cause that might be operating to bring about the behavioral abnormality. The starting point should be a change to the *Correct Nutrition* regimen detailed in Chapter II, which eliminates caffeine, chemicals used in processed foods and refined sugar. It also prevents constipation and assures the rapid elimination of body waste with the noxious substances contained within it.

Prevention and Treatment of The Hyperactive Child Syndrome

1. The *Correct Nutrition* regimen as detailed in Chapter II, coupled with an exercise program can cause tremendous improvement and marked behavioral changes for the better in *The Hyperactive Child*.

CHAPTER XX

Halitosis

"We are what we eat." Our diets will in great measure determine the extent to which we are afflicted with "bad breath" or repulsive "body odor". When the diabetic is in severe acidosis, we can smell the acetone breath, often from across a room. The odoriferous or fetid breath of the uremic patient is characteristic, and the inebriated alcoholic seems to reek of alcohol from the breath and body as well.

"Halitosis" means bad breath, and we may have an offensive breath, even though our teeth are clean and healthy, and our mouths and nasal passages are free from disease. The foul odor may come from the lungs, and no breath freshener, breath deodorant, or mouthwash will have any effect other than to temporarily cover it up or overpower it with a different and less noxious scent.

Most bad breath or "halitosis" can be prevented by the correct nutrition regimen detailed in Chapter II, but the diet must be adhered to religiously in all aspects and complete cure is usually not effected until most of any excessive weight has been eliminated.

Body Odor

May I reiterate, "We are what we eat". "Body odor" is in some respects unique, but diet has a great influence on both the quality and the quantity of the odor radiating from the body surface.

Even some of the Indian tribes, living on the Great Plains in centuries past, were aware of the effects of food on body odor. They knew that horses had an acute sense of smell; and in order to capture wild horses, they knew that they must be as odor-free as possible. They would abstain from eating any fat, fish, or meat for long periods of time, existing for weeks on roots, herbs, grains, and berries before trying to trap and capture wild horses. They were also known to employ these dietary precautions before going on the "warpath" or on raiding forays, in order not to betray their presence to the dogs in enemy camps.

When our sweat glands and sebaceous glands secrete, they are shedding desquamating cells and products of body metabolism. We can change the quality of some of the malodorous portions of these secretions by changing our diets to the nutrition regimen detailed in Chapter II.

Many people turn to the so called "breath fresheners", "breath deodorants", "mouthwashes", "antiperspirants" and "odor eaters" to mask the offensive body odors that are actually due in large part to their high-sugar, high-fat, low-fiber diets.

The safer, more natural and healthful approach to prevention of offensive body and foot odors is correct nutrition as detailed in Chapter II.

Prevention and Treatment of Halitosis and Offensive Body Odor

1. The *Correct Nutrition* regimen as detailed in Chapter II, which allows *no* refined carbohydrates (especially sugar, white rice and white flour) and *no* alcoholic beverages and which stresses the consumption of large quantities of fresh, raw or steamed vegetables and fresh, raw fruit, is the number one priority.
2. Loss of excess weight is the second priority.
3. The *Exercise Program* detailed in Chapter III is the third priority.

Cigarettes

We are all familiar with the warning "*Cigarette Smoking* may be *Harmful* to your *Health"*, and we should probably deal with some specific instances rather than let this generality slip by with too little attention.

The most important association of cigarette smoking with disease is probably its relation to atherosclerosis, a degenerative disease causing narrowing and clogging of the arteries, especially those nourishing the heart and brain. Disease of these vessels is responsible for most deaths from "heart disease" and "stroke". "Cancer of the lung", "cancer of the urinary bladder", and "emphysema" are three other "killers" that have been listed as related to cigarette smoking, and the danger of birth defects must be considered in those smoking during pregnancy. Tissue hypoxia may be a causative factor in all of the above in addition to the chemical irritation. Tissue hypoxia means that too little oxygen is getting to the tissue cells of the body to keep them functioning in a normal, healthy manner. When individuals smoke, or breathe someone else's smoke, they take in chemical poisons, including carbon monoxide which is a colorless, odorless, tasteless and non-irritating gas that is a product of combustion or burning. This carbon monoxide is drawn into the lungs, dissolves into the blood, and quickly combines with the hemoglobin of the red blood cells, rendering them less capable or incapable of carrying oxygen. The affinity of carbon monoxide for hemoglobin is 200 times that of oxygen, and therefore can prevent the red cell from picking up oxygen to take to the tissues. This causes the tissue hypoxia or suffocation damage to the body cells.

Alcohol

Ethyl "alcohol" is the active ingredient of beer, wine, whiskey, gin, ale and brandy; and it is a drug, just as are heroin, cocaine, marijuana and LSD. Those alcoholic beverages with the higher percentages of alcohol contain in addition, ethers for taste and several impurities such as amyl alcohol (fusel oil) and acetaldehyde, which act the same as alcohol but are more toxic or poisonous.

"Alcohol" is omitted in a good nutrition program, because it provides calories but nothing else of value such as fiber or significant amounts of vitamins or minerals. In addition to having nothing to recommend it, alcohol can have very serious, life-threatening consequences in addition to alcoholism and nutritional deficiencies. Alcohol raises the triglyceride and uric acid levels in the blood producing hyperlipidemia and hyperuricemia. Hyperlipidemia is a risk factor for coronary heart disease, and hyperuricemia for gouty arthritis. Alcohol also causes gastritis (inflammation of the stomach), liver disease, polyneuritis, and central nervous system damage. Alcoholic beverages have also been implicated as causative of birth defects and other problems related to infant morbidity and mortality.

Caffeine

"Caffeine" and other xanthine derivatives are found in coffee, tea, cocoa, chocolate and many of the carbonated soft drinks. Caffeine is suspect as causative of birth defects and peptic ulcer. As we all know, caffeine can produce insomnia (sleeplessness), and it intensifies the problem of the "hyperactive child". Perhaps the most dangerous and least appreciated complications of caffeine-use in susceptible individuals are cardiac arrhythmias (irregular heart beats and tachycardias).

CHAPTER XXI

Conclusions

We have discussed a host of diseases, many seemingly unrelated, which are preventable, and some even curable, by means of a combination of correct nutrition and exercise programs alone. We could add other diseases to this list and make a very strong case for their acceptance. Among these is the "Common Cold". This virus infection seems unable to make any impression on the individuals who follow this nutrition and exercise program. Apparently the natural resistance becomes so strong that the organisms cannot prevail against the defenses of the healthy body.

In light of this knowledge, there are certain Public Health programs which should probably be instituted.

1. Preschool, kindergarten and elementary school teachers should be encouraged to teach "nutrition" and "exercise" as a major part of their programs.
2. School cafeterias should probably serve only skim milk, fresh fruits, fresh vegetables, legumes and whole-grain cereals and breads. Refined sugars and products made with refined sugars should be barred.
3. School vending machines should probably be allowed to dispense only skim milk and fresh fruits.
4. Prisons, jails and other similar public institutions should probably be mandated to serve only this physical-health and mental-health promoting diet, and exercise programs should be encouraged. Attendance (though not participation) should probably be compulsory at daily exercise sessions.

5. Hospital patients on "General Diet" should be on this nutrition program, both for health and educational reasons; and those patients, who are capable, should be started on appropriate exercise programs.

6. The "Nursing Homes" and "Senior Citizen Homes" are outstanding examples of neglect of "correct" nutrition and adequate exercise programs. "Good" food and "good" nutrition are probably the rule, but "correct" nutrition with regular, relatively strenuous exercise programs designed to meet the unique needs of each individual are definitely not the rule. To allow old people to sit around all day without planned, relatively strenuous physical exercise, encourages disuse atrophy of muscles, limitation of motion of joints and osteoporosis. To feed these elderly people a diet high in refined sugar, fat and fried foods can lead only to a furthering of their atherosclerosis and their progress down the road to senility.

If the above programs were instituted, the nutrition and physical fitness awareness level would rise quickly and dramatically. Much of the public would recognize benefits to be derived by compliance and the risks faced by non-compliance. They would then tend to make educated choices rather than blind ones and the cost of medical care might conceivably plunge downward.

GLOSSARY

Achilles tendon: the strong, thick tendon connecting the posterior calf muscles to the heel bone (calcaneus).

acne: an inflammatory disease of the skin characterized by eruptions, especially on the face.

afflictions: diseases or maladies or illnesses.

Alzheimer's Disease: an organic dementia (see dementia), usually beginning in persons under 50 years of age. It is also called presenile dementia.

anal canal: the terminal portion of the intestinal tract (only a little over one inch long) between the rectum and the anal opening.

androgenic hormones: male hormones.

anesthetic: an agent that has reversible effects and one that depresses nerve cell function with decrease or loss of sensation.

aneurysm: a circumscribed dilation of an artery, or a blood containing tumor connected to an artery.

angina: in this context, it refers to chest pain on exertion due to insufficient blood supply to the heart.

aorta: the largest artery in the body. It extends from the heart, through the chest and abdomen, to about one inch below the level of the umbilicus or belly-button.

arrhythmia: an irregularity in the rate or rhythm of the heartbeat.

arteriosclerosis: often referred to as "hardening of the arteries". Atherosclerosis is one form of arteriosclerosis.

artery: a blood vessel carrying oxygenated blood from the heart to the tissues and organs of the body. The pulmonary artery to the lungs is the only artery carrying deoxygenated blood.

arthritis: inflammation of the joints.

arthropathy: joint disease where inflammation is not a major factor.

atherosclerosis: a form of arteriosclerosis with atheromatous plaque formation in arterial walls causing constriction of the lumen and decrease in blood flow.

atrophy: a wasting away of a tissue or organ due to defective nutrition or disuse.

β-cells: these are specialized pancreatic cells which produce insulin.

calcification: in this context, calcification refers to the deposition of calcium salts, bone-like material, in the walls of arteries.

caliber: the diameter or the circumference.

calorie: a unit of heat or energy content of a food.

carbohydrates: these are the sugars and starches. They yield about 4 calories of energy to the gram.

cardiac: pertaining to the heart.

caries, dental: see dental caries.

cerebral thrombosis: this refers to the clotting of blood in a cerebral or brain artery, thus occluding the artery and stopping the blood flow to a portion of the brain.

cerebrovascular: this simply means brain blood vessels. A cerebrovascular disease would be one involving blood vessels to the brain.

cholelithiasis: gallstones.

cholesterol: this is one of the blood lipids. The cholesterol level in the blood should be below 150 to ensure that atheromatous plaque is not forming in blood vessel walls.

colon: this is the large intestine and it extends from the small intestine to the anal canal.

colonic loading: an abnormal filling of the large bowel or colon caused by constipation with stagnation and sludging of intestinal contents.

colonic stasis: sludging and stagnation of fecal material in the large bowel or colon.

coronary arteries: the arteries in the walls of the heart that nourish the heart.

degeneration: (as in degenerative diseases, degenerative arthritis and joint degeneration). This signifies deterioration or pathologic change in cells or tissues, impairing or destroying their functions.

dementia: general mental deterioration.

dental caries: decay or destruction of teeth.

diabetes mellitus: sugar diabetes.

diaphragm: this refers to the musculotendinous wall separating the chest cavity from the abdominal cavity.

disuse atrophy: a wasting away of a tissue or organ from disuse.

diverticulitis: inflammation of a diverticulum or of diverticula.

diverticulosis: a condition or disease where diverticula are found.

diverticulum: in this context, it is a small sac or pouch caused by abnormally high pressures within the large bowel (colon). The plural of diverticulum is diverticula.

dowager's hump: a humpback condition in postmenopausal women. It is caused by fracture of vertebral bodies due to osteoporosis. It is frequently painless.

duodenum: the C-shaped portion of the small intestine into which the stomach empties. It is the upper portion of the small intestine.

epidemiology: the study of the prevalence and distribution of disease.

estrogenic hormone: female hormone.

fiber: the undigestible portion of the cell walls of fruits, vegetables, legumes and whole grains.

fracture: a break, especially the breaking of a bone.

gangrene: death of tissue due to diminished or insufficient blood supply.

gastrointestinal tract: the alimentary canal or the pathway for food from the mouth to the anus.

glossary: a list of difficult, basic technical terms with definitions.

glucose: a sugar.

gout: a recurrent acute arthritis of sudden onset associated with hyperuricemia (high blood levels of uric acid).

hemoglobin: the red protein of red blood cells that transports oxygen.

hemorrhoids: dilated veins in the anal canal, usually caused by straining during bowel movements.

hernia: the protrusion of a part or structure through the tissues normally containing it.

hiatus: an opening, a foramen, an aperture or a fissure.

hormones: chemical substances formed in one organ or part of the body and carried by the blood stream to influence another organ or part.

hyperglycemia: an abnormally high concentration of glucose (sugar) in the blood.

hyperlipidemia: an abnormally high concentration of lipids (fats) in the blood.

hyperuricemia: an abnormally high concentration of uric acid in the blood.

hypoglycemia: an abnormally low concentration of glucose (sugar) in the blood.

hypoglycemic drugs: drugs which tend to lower the concentration of glucose (sugar) in the blood.

hypopituitarism: a condition caused by diminished activity of the anterior lobe of the pituitary gland.

hypothalamus: a region of the brain.

hypothyroidism: diminished production of thyroid hormone by the thyroid gland.

hypoxia: abnormally low levels of oxygen in the blood or tissues.

iatric: caused by medicine or by a physician.

iatrogenic: denoting an unfavorable response to therapy, or induced by the therapy itself.

infarction: tissue damage due to sudden insufficiency of arterial supply (see myocardial infarction).

insulin: a hormone, secreted by the β-cells of the pancreas, which promotes the utilization of glucose (sugar).

intraluminal pressure: in this context, it refers to the abnormally high pressures in the large intestine (colon) which tend to balloon-out the walls with the formation of small outpouchings or sacs called diverticula.

ischemia: inadequate blood supply.

lipids: substances which are fat-soluble (included are fatty acids, triglycerides, cholesterol, etc.).

loading: see colonic loading.

"Maintenance Level": the caloric intake that maintains weight without significant gain or loss as one carries out the daily routines.

malady: a disease or affliction or illness.

malignancy: in this context, it means cancer (see malignant).

malignant: having the properties of being destructive and invasive and having the ability to metastasize and spread (cancerous).

menopause: termination of the menstrual life.

morbidity: a state of being diseased or ill.

mortality: in this context, it means death rate.

myocardial infarction: a sudden insufficiency of the arterial blood supply to a region of the myocardium (the muscular walls of the heart). The ischemic or infarcted region may become necrotic.

necrosis: death of cells or tissue.

necrotic: pertaining to necrosis.

obesity: excessively fat.

occult: hidden or concealed.

orthopedic: in this context, the medical specialty concerned with the treatment of diseases of the bones and other supporting structures.

osteoporosis: reduction in the quantity of bone or atrophy of skeletal tissue.
a disease characterized by a demineralization of bone.

palliative: treatment which may alleviate symptoms but does not cure the disease.

pancreas: the abdominal organ which, among other functions, produces the hormone, insulin.

pectinate line: the line in the anal canal where the mucosa of the bowel meets the skin.

peptic ulcer: peptic means pertaining to the stomach, and an ulcer is a lesion or wound with destruction of surface tissues. However, peptic ulcers are most frequently found in the duodenum, but they occur in the stomach and elsewhere.

peritonitis: inflammation or infection of the inner lining of the abdominal cavity.

plaque: in this context, an atheromatous lesion in a blood vessel wall causing narrowing of the blood channel.

proprietary: in this context, a medicine or drug that can be purchased without a prescription.

prostate: a male sex gland found at the base of the urinary bladder.

pruritus ani: itching in the anal region.

pulmonary: pertaining to the lung.

pulmonary embolus: a blood clot that lodges in the lung.

rectum: that portion of the large intestine (colon) between the sigmoid portion of the colon and the anal canal.

regression: in this context, a return toward normal from the diseased state.

rheumatism: a common term for the affliction characterized by pain, tenderness and stiffness of muscles and structures surrounding the joints.

sebaceous glands: glands in the skin which secrete sebum, a fatty oily substance.

senile dementia: mental deterioration of the aged usually due to atherosclerosis.

senility: physical and mental deterioration in the aged, hastened by lack of proper nutrition and regular, relatively strenuous physical exercise programs.

sequelae: morbid conditions following as a consequence of a disease.

stasis: see colonic stasis.

"stroke": a lay term denoting a sudden neurological affliction, usually related to decreased blood supply to the brain.

tendonitis: inflammation of a tendon.

thrombosis: a clotting of blood within a blood vessel.

trauma: an injury.

triglycerides: certain lipids found in the blood.

ulcer: a lesion on the surface of the skin or on the mucous membrane lining of the mouth, stomach, intestines, etc. There is usually tissue destruction and inflammation.

varicocele: abnormally enlarged dilated veins in the scrotal sac of the male. These veins drain the testicle.

varicose veins: enlarged, dilated veins.

vascular: pertaining to blood vessels.

vein: a blood vessel that conveys blood toward the heart.

"Western" diet: the high-fat, low-fiber diet prevalent in the "Western" world.

"Western" world: Europe and the United States and Canada.

INDEX

—————D—————

—————E—————

—————F—————